It's A Fit!

DRESSING WITH STYLE, COMFORT AND CONFIDENCE

Susan Graver

DRESSING WITH
STYLE, COMFORT
AND CONFIDENCE

It's A Fit!

Susan Graver

QVC'S FASHION DESIGNER

QVC PUBLISHING, INC.

QVC Publishing, Inc.
Jill Cohen, Vice President and Publisher
Ellen Bruzelius, General Manager
Sarah Butterworth, Editorial Director
Karen Murgolo, Director of Rights and Acquisitions
Cassandra Reynolds, Publishing Assistant

Produced in association with Patrick Filley Associates, Inc. and
Hermitage Publishing Services
Design, Debra Drodvillo/Notion Studio
Illustrations by Mary Lynn Blasutta
Photography by William Rutledge and Mark Thomas

QVC Publishing books are available at special discounts when purchased
in bulk for premiums and sales promotions as well as for fund-raising or
educational use. Special editions or book excerpts can be created to
specification. For details, contact QVC Publishing, 50 Main Street, Suite
201, Mt. Kisco, NY 10549.

Published by QVC Publishing, Inc., 50 Main Street, Mt. Kisco, NY 10549

Manufactured in U.S.A.

ISBN: 1-928998-38-0

First Edition
10 9 8 7 6 5 4 3 2 1

Dedication

My family is first and foremost in my life: my husband, Richard, and my three wonderful children, Michael, David, and Jaclyn. They are the wind beneath my wings. They inspire my values, my goals, and my accomplishments. Richard has supported me throughout my career, encouraging me and urging me on with his love, patience, and wisdom. I look to him for emotional support, business advice, and even advice on what to wear—he always knows what looks most flattering on me! Richard is my very best friend, and my children are my truest blessing. This book is dedicated to them.

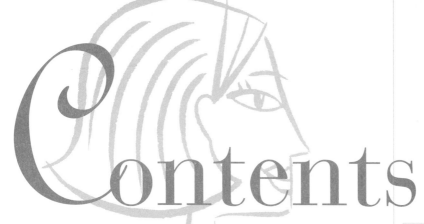

Contents

$\mathcal{I}$ntroduction

I almost called this book, "Susan Graver: Always Rushing", because like most of you, I am a woman constantly on the go. I am always shopping for new, up-to-the-minute designs; I oversee a dedicated staff of artists and pattern makers; I meet with buyers; I host a TV show—and I make sure I save time for what's most important in my life: my husband Richard and my three terrific children Michael, David, and Jaclyn. Of course when we're relaxing together, we're always hiking or playing golf or tennis or skiing. So even when I'm not working, I'm still rushing! You and I both know that an active lifestyle puts a huge strain on any woman's wardrobe. We need clothes that can do double, sometimes triple, duty—taking us from the office to a night out—clothes that are easy to care for and yet fresh and stylish.

In this book, I'm going to help you build a wardrobe based on your lifestyle, your body type, and your personality, but there will be only one surefire way to tell if we've succeeded: do your clothes make you feel confident? If your closet is full of dowdy, out-of-style shirts and slacks, if your skirts are too tight or your blouses faded, you're going to feel it when you step out into the world. You might be as qualified as the next person for that job, but that little nagging doubt, that little slump in your shoulders, will keep you from getting what you want. You may also learn that sometimes less is more. Your wardrobe may be overcrowded and cluttered with useless items that are keeping you from seeing clearly and finding neat, clean pieces that work best for you. In this book I will teach you how to dress fashionably for your lifestyle. Dressing easily and comfortably without spending a fortune. I am a firm believer in "You are only as pretty as you feel." I believe you should dress in outfits that work for you. I am not going to dictate what fashion is in style or not, but I will help you learn to look your best in what fits you and your lifestyle. I do not go for cookie-cutter looks. I think that fashion should be very personal—it should enhance one's personality, bringing out one's own beauty.

I remember when I was fourteen or fifteen, I was invited to a party and I wanted the perfect outfit. I went from store to store, searching every rack, but I just couldn't find anything I liked. So I decided to make my own outfit. I picked out the fabric. I sketched the design. I worked day and night to get it just right. In the end, I was thrilled with my creation: a white satin jumpsuit. Looking back, it was so over the top! But it didn't matter, I loved it. Would I wear that jumpsuit today? Honestly, I'd have to say no. But did it make me *feel* beautiful then? Indisputably, yes. I felt gorgeous and proud and confident. So was that piece of clothing a success? Most definitely.

Confidence is the one thing I don't think I can stress enough. Your clothes should make you look and feel great. It's the designer's job to create well-made, gorgeous, great-fitting garments, and it's your job to know yourself, your style, and your daily needs well enough to choose the pieces that are right for you. Every one of us has a piece of clothing in her closet that corresponds to my white satin jumpsuit. A special outfit that makes us feel stunning. But let's face it, how often is that white satin jumpsuit appropriate? Are you really going to wear it to a business meeting, on a lunch date, or to pick up your kids from school? My goal in writing this book is to help you select versatile pieces to create outfits that will look great on you—no matter what your size or body shape—and let you feel fabulous about yourself 365 days a year.

So enjoy!

Susan Graver

Who Am

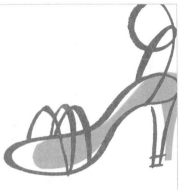

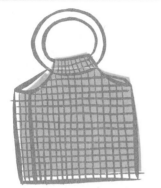

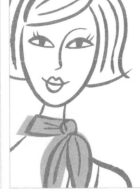

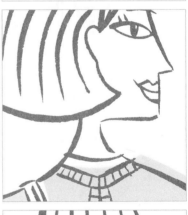

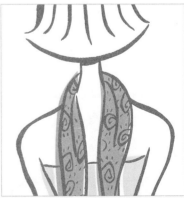

Chapter 1

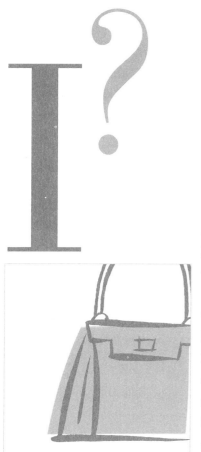

Since we're going to spend most of this book helping you get to know yourself, it's only fair that you get to know me and a little of what I do.

Fashion and design have been such a large part of my life for so long, I can't imagine doing anything else. I think I've developed a lot of insights over the years, and I'm thrilled to have the chance to share them with you.

I guess it was inevitable I would find a home on QVC, where I've spent twelve wonderful years presenting my creations, because as a girl my passions were art, fashion, and performing. I loved to draw and paint. My mother remembers one of my drawings from kindergarten. It was a self-portrait. When you turned the paper over, I had drawn the back of myself as well. She knew right then and there that I had a unique way of expressing myself—and that I couldn't stand to leave things half done!

As a kid, I spent hours playing with my Barbie and making beautiful outfits for her. When I was fifteen my parents bought me my own sewing machine. I taught myself how to make patterns and sew, and I began creating clothes for myself. I remember designing a beautiful suit with covered buttons in a soft, fluid fabric; it was a peplum jacket over a slim skirt. I made halter tops out of scarves attached to shoelaces or old necklaces.

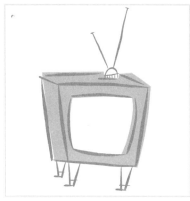

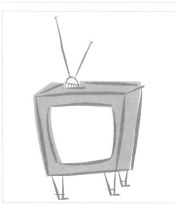

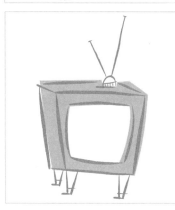

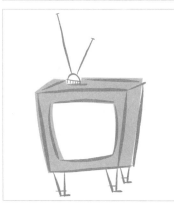

And wouldn't you know it, I recently saw a halter-top in a fashion magazine from an expensive, posh designer. Mine were just as beautiful and cost next to nothing! Even back then, I had a very independent sense of style. It didn't matter what everyone else was wearing—I knew what *I* liked and what *I* wanted to wear. I especially loved dresses and clothes made from luxurious fabrics. I was no tomboy that's for sure. I loved frills and fancy decoration, anything that made a piece really stand out.

In addition to expressing myself in fashion, I also loved performing and singing. I had a wonderful, warm family. Most weekends we would go to my grandmother's house, where I would entertain her neighbors on the front stoop, singing and dancing, performing little numbers my mom choreographed for me. I was such a ham! Now, years later, I've found a way to marry my two great loves—I get to design great clothes and then bring them to you on my own TV show!

When I graduated from college, I was headed toward a career in either the visual arts or show business. My soon-to-be in-laws were in the garment industry and suggested that since I was so outgoing and artistic, fashion might be the perfect combination of art and performing I was looking for. I think it was Audrey Graver, my mother-in-law, who suggested I take myself down to 1407 Seventh Avenue (one of the two biggest, most famous fashion buildings in New York) and find out who was hiring. The garment district, an area in midtown Manhattan where most of America's major designers have their showrooms, is a bustling part of town full of double-parked trucks unloading rolling racks of clothes, anything from the most outlandish studded jeans to the most respectable Harris-tweed suits. All the sights and sounds and rushing people overwhelmed me; but I was invigorated too. I knew I belonged there, with all those rushing people.

I figured with all the coming and going, who would better know what was going on than the elevator operator? So I marched up to the man who worked the elevator and asked if he knew of anyone hiring. What a nerve! The "all-knowing" elevator operator laughed and told me, in fact, that he had just heard of a designer who had left a big firm to start her own business. He was sure she was looking for people.

I thanked him, called the designer, and sure enough, I was hired right away as her Girl Friday. I did every sort of job around the office you can imagine. While it wasn't what I ultimately wanted, it got me in the door. Within a few months I landed a new job with a fast-growing company, where I stayed for close to ten years and eventually learned enough to open my own design studio in the heart of the garment district of Manhattan.

Inside the Graver Studio

Though I'm the one on television, there is an incredibly dedicated team behind the Susan Graver label. Most of the people working for me today have been with me since I first struck out on my own. I've already mentioned Audrey Graver, my mother-in-law, who is dynamic and has a keen eye for fashion. She is full of energy and makes things happen. Together we shop and scout trends, come up with colors and prints, and choose fabrics and styles. Audrey and I are such great friends, it's almost too much fun coming into work. We're both Sagittarians, and we literally finish each other's sentences. Audrey worked in the fashion industry with my father-in-law, Jack Graver for several years doing sales and design. She joined me after his retirement and we've been a team ever since. It's incredible how often we're on exactly the same page when it comes to styles and trends. It's as if we can read each other's minds.

Audrey and I could have all the great ideas in the world but if we didn't have a fabulous staff to put our ideas into production, none of it would matter. Betty Mui and Joanne Cheung, my patternmakers, have both been with me for over ten years.

Both studied at FIT (The Fashion Institute of Technology in New York.) They are the ones who transform our design ideas into garments. Their contribution is a very important part of the business. Two of the best seamstresses around, Nelly Escobar and Germania Mercier, construct samples from the patterns either Betty or Joanne has created. Later, we'll have a model try it on to make sure it looks great on a real person.

Ann Zachariades, my office manager, has been with me for over seven years. She studied fashion merchandising. She now runs the showroom, answers the phone, handles the bills, and oversees customer relations.

Ann and Betty

"Besides running the showroom, I also sort the fan mail," Ann laughs. "Susan gets a hundred to two hundred fan letters a week, and she reads every single one. They ask Susan for advice on color and prints. It's especially fun when the fans include photos. We keep an album of them.

Susan is such a pleasure to work with. She comes in and she's always happy. Though I'm sure she's had as many bad days as the rest of us, you'd never imagine it from the way she is around the office. She keeps us upbeat and she makes us feel really good about ourselves. What you see on television is exactly how she is."

"It's like a family around here," Betty says. "This was my second job out of the Fashion Institute, and I can't imagine being anywhere else. We eat lunch together every day, we throw great birthday parties. I sometimes have more fun at work than I do at home!"

Superfan Shirley

A few years ago, I received a phone call from a woman named Shirley who had recently been in the hospital. She was a huge fan, and during her hospital stay, her husband brought in her Susan Graver clothing and hung it all around her room. Shirley said that just looking at the clothes and thinking about where she was going to wear them when she got out gave her something to live for. Shirley has called regularly over the last few years to critique my shows. Her advice is always heartfelt and we have become friends.

The Journey of a Blouse

It's a long and wonderful journey from the conception of a garment until it makes its way into your closet. Let's look at the life of a single blouse, from inspiration, through production, to its television debut on my show. You will get an overview of how the fashion industry works, without ever leaving your house.

Our blouse begins at least six months before you ever see it, at the very first design phase of each season. I begin each season's line by putting together two or three large "trend boards." These are collages of pictures that identify what I believe to be the fashion-forward trends for the new season. The design of our shirt will grow out of this research—from my shopping trips around New York, visits to Europe, and from looking through the best of the fashion magazines. I usually do three trend boards: one for colors, one for fabrics, and one for fashion trends. For example, when I was working on Fall 2000, I saw deep reds, a range of greens, and lots of winter whites as the colors coming in for fall. With fabrics, I saw that skins had become very fashionable—pony skin, suede, leather—as well as soft, fleecy yarns. In the fashion trends category, I saw that capes and ponchos were all the rage, as were garments with lots of embroidery, embellishment, and trimming. So when I was designing our blouse, I kept our classic lines in mind, but incorporated some of what I had identified as new and exciting. The challenge is to design a garment that can be integrated into your classic wardrobe but still says "today."

At the same time that I'm pulling together pictures for the trend boards, I'm meeting with fabric designers, who present their ideas in paintings. I work with these artists, suggesting they lighten a color here or enlarge an element, such as a paisley, there, until we get exactly the look I'm going for. Audrey is always very involved at this stage. All in all, it's a very collaborative process. We show the paintings around the office and get a general consensus before presenting them to QVC. Out of twenty-five to thirty designs, we usually choose twenty-four or so to anchor the new season's line.

After the designs are ready, we "shop" the fabrics. (Actually, Audrey and I are always shopping fabric lines, it's an ongoing process.) Representatives from textile mills stop into the showroom with books of samples. It's very important to marry texture with design, color, and weight. You might not want a very light print on a thick, bulky fabric. Likewise, a big, geometric print might overwhelm something sheer. When I've decided which fabric is perfect for each print, it's sent to the mill where samples are "struck off". This is a complicated process in which the pattern is applied to the fabric. The sample comes back for my approval as well as QVC's approval. Over half the time, I have to send it back because the color is not quite right, or the design isn't crisp enough, or the print needs to be reduced or cleaned up. Since the whole season's collection will be developed around these prints, they have to be perfect before the strike-off phase is over.

About this time I present the trend boards, sketches, examples of garments I've bought, fabric samples, and the fabric paintings to the buyers at QVC. I've done my research and identified what I think are the biggest trends in the upcoming season, but my buyers and I still need to put our heads together. There is always the chance that I've identified pink as the hot new color and they've identified orange. Usually we totally agree from the start, although once in a while our ideas are different. When this happens my trend boards can really help because they're like a mini-encyclopedia of the latest colors, fabrics, and looks.

During this big meeting, we make a final decision on my line for the coming season. Based on their knowledge of what other QVC designers are doing, the buyers choose a group of garments from the designs I've presented. Occasionally, I'll fight to include a piece or a print that the buyers haven't chosen—often because it's close to something in another QVC designer's line. Sometimes I win, sometimes I lose, but most of the choices are joint decisions. I try to be pragmatic. I want my line to be new and different, and I don't want duplicate designs that are already out there. There is no point in two designers offering pieces that are practically the same. We want each line to be unique, and it's the buyers' job to see the big picture.

Once the buyers and I have agreed on the collection, I order larger quantities of the fabrics we've chosen from my manufacturers. We then have samples of each garment in the correct print and fabric made for final approval. There is still time to change our minds, and occasionally we do just that. Not long ago I designed a whimsical little print and we used it for a jacket. Once we saw the jacket made up, it seemed too structured for the fabric. The buyer and I both decided the print would work much better for a sundress. Seeing samples—and not just blindly ordering a huge quantity of any design—is a crucial step because every once in a while we end up avoiding what would be a real disaster.

Once we see the sample and give your blouse the go-ahead, the manufacturer makes up the ordered quantity, which is shipped to the QVC warehouse. Then comes the very best part for me. I get to present it live on air.

My Design Philosophy

For me, designing is a sixth sense. It's a feeling of what will be strong for the upcoming season. One of my most important fashion statements was made back in 1989 when the market was heavily promoting large floral prints and cabbage-rose motifs. I decided to keep my designs clean, with positive/negative contrasting black and white dots. It was simple, fresh, and new looking. Bloomingdales catalog featured my line and it was a huge success. Many other major department stores and specialty chains followed suit. A knowledge of what the market is doing and what the trends are in Europe where things happen first is important. But I design from my own gut. I design with my own sense of what is right and what is most beautiful and flattering to women of all walks of life.

A Day at QVC

It's 4:30 a.m. and I'm kissing my husband good-bye. Another man is waiting for me in a car outside and my suitcase is by the door. No, I'm not walking out on my family, it's just a typical Thursday morning and I'm off to QVC to do my 9:00 a.m. show. I can depend upon my driver Al (Hector Alfonso) who has been getting up by 3:00 a.m. for over eight years to drive me the three hours from my house to the QVC studio. It's tough starting the day so early, but I want to be able to spend as much time with my family as I can, and the only other choice would be to sleep every Wednesday night away from home.

Before long, we're pulling into Studio Park, where QVC has a huge complex of offices, studios, and shops—and a great commissary. I make my way past the sound stages, where In the Kitchen with Bob and The Morning Show are shot, to my dressing room. There, Gina Francesco, my makeup artist, does my makeup and hair. She's been with me for over nine years and knows all my likes and dislikes. I often ask her advice about what shoes and accessories I should pair with the outfit I'll be wearing on the air. Gina studied art and eventually took up the family business of makeup design. She's taught me most of what I know about cosmetics and hair. As she puts on my foundation and rolls my hair, I drink my first cup of coffee and slowly start to wake up. I try not to think about what I'm going to say on air, because I never want to sound scripted. I think that's the biggest reason I'm so relaxed when I get in front of the camera—I just let whatever wants to come out, come out. If I were trying to remember what to say, it would probably sound phony. And I'd be far more nervous!

The green room where I get dressed and wait to go on air is really nice. It's set up like a small apartment with a kitchenette and a living room. There is a big comfortable sofa and a TV tuned to QVC so that I can watch what's on before me. I look for "Today's Special Value". It's usually something I'd love to have! I watch to see if Pat DeMentri is on The Morning Show because I love working with her. She is such a warm and wonderful person, I truly enjoy and look forward to my hour with her. Although all the other hosts are also terrific to work with, Pat is special to me. I also like to check out how Pat looks, since she is always wearing one of my outfits.

Pat DeMentri, Susan's Co-host

"I absolutely adore Susan," Pat DeMentri says. "We did our very first show together about ten years ago, and since then we've become the best of friends. We've shared each other's ups and downs; our children have grown up together. Neither of us has a lot of time outside of work, so we pack more socializing into an hour than most women do in a week.

"Our show together is my last show of the day— I've been up since three in the morning and sometimes I feel like I'm going to drop, but Susan always perks me right up. There is never a day that she comes in that she's not excited and energized. Even though we can't see the viewers out there, we know they come back every single week and they share our lives. I love to see how Susan has evolved and how she's responded to the customers through their calls and letters. It's really fun for me—I love fashion and I get to shop along with the viewers.

"Susan does so much for us women today, who are stressed and who need to watch our pennies. She's one of us. She knows what it's like to get up early and be a mom and have to look good. She knows what we need, and she makes us feel like a million bucks."

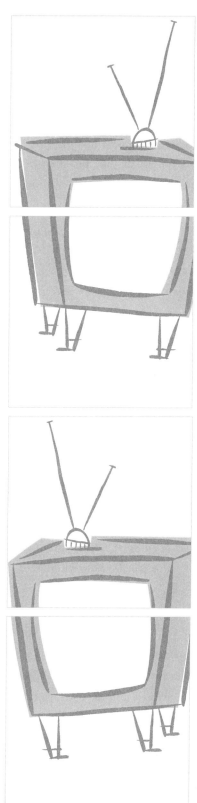

About half an hour before we go on air, Liana Mattera who works as a coordinator between QVC and my manufacturer, brings me the outfit I'm going to wear and tells me how the models are doing. The day before the show, I am always given what is called a PAL sheet—don't ask me what that stands for! It's a list of all the outfits the models are going to be wearing, and in what order. The PAL sheet lets me make sure both the outfits and models are shown to their best advantage. I can pick the combinations I prefer and suggest the pieces that shouldn't be worn together. I also check the shoes, hose, and accessories that the models will be wearing. Everything has to be done in advance since the show is live. I've been working with the same models for years and we've become great friends. I know I can count on them to look great—one less thing to worry about before we go on camera.

After I get into my clothes (the clothing is brought to me right before the show—no time to hem or fix), I am hooked up with an IFB (interrupt feedback) pack. This is a little device that hooks onto my waistband under whatever top I'm wearing. It's attached to a long cord with a miniature earphone that runs up under my top and tucks in my left ear. They usually tape the cord to the back of my neck so that it doesn't show. The IFB pack is so small, most viewers never know I'm wearing it. Through the earphone I can hear the producers while we're on air, telling me when commercial breaks are almost over, what items are sold out—things like that. I also hear the callers through this little earphone. At first it was weird having a little voice in my ear all the time, but now I'm totally used to it. Besides the IFB pack, they also clip a microphone pack to my waistband and run a tiny microphone up the front of my top and out at my collar.

Once I'm all rigged up, I make my way to the sound-stage. I pass behind other sets and the racks of clothes that have been carefully prepared for the day's show. Pat (or one of the other hosts) introduces me and I join her on my own sofa with colorful peachskin pillows. I just love being live on air. I'm always so energized by presenting my clothes, talking to the viewers, and hearing their feedback. It's the best! I've been asked a hundred times, "How can you talk for an hour, or even two hours, about your clothes? How can you think of that much to say?" All I can tell you is that it comes so easily. As a matter of fact I am so energized when I'm on the air that I sometimes wonder if my excitement makes me talk too much! Because I'm the designer—I'm not just a celebrity host with no connection to the product—I know these clothes inside and out. I, along with my team, created them. I've been involved in every step of the process that went into making them (and now, so have you!). I don't have to struggle to remember details about each item because I've lived with them through the entire design and manufacturing cycle. And I'm always excited about passing on a great value, so I think my enthusiasm just takes over.

It's interesting, the difference between what you see on TV and what we see sitting in front of the camera. We have at least four cameras trained on us at all times and two TV monitors to watch. One monitor, called the on-line monitor, shows what is currently being broadcast, so that we can see the garment we're holding as it looks on air or the stills we're presenting. The other monitor, called the preview monitor, shows what shot the cameramen are setting up next. These monitors are especially important for the production coordinator. They're also important for the person who has the job of sneaking on and off the set with the racks of clothes we're showing you. If we're done showing trousers, he'll whisk them away and replace them with skirts. The trick for him is to get on and off the set while the cameras are showing something else. So he watches both the on-line and preview monitors to make sure he doesn't get caught. Some of the funniest moments I've had on air are times when he didn't make it, or accidentally bumped a garment into me as he ran off stage. It's a carefully coordinated procedure, but being live, you never know when something could go wrong.

Pat and I present the garments for that show, a selection of new designs and old favorites. We get updates in our ears about which items are low in stock and which sizes have sold out. The time seems to fly by. Sometimes we look up and wave at a studio tour passing by. They can watch us through a big window at the back of the studio. That's always fun. But really, I think my favorite part of any show is talking to the viewers. I just love to hear what they have to say and what ideas they have for new items. I never take my audience for granted. It's like throwing a

Behind the Scenes with Susan's Models

Backstage, the models' dressing room is set up with lighted mirrors and racks of clothes. Susan works with six models, most of whom have been with her for years: Iris, Karen, Maria, Lisa, Ginger, and Sioux. They arrive half an hour before the show starts to do their own hair and makeup.

The fashion coordinator who will work the show is usually at work by 2:00 a.m. the night before Susan goes on at 9:00 a.m. She lines up the clothes that are to be modeled, presses them, and sometimes sets up the still shots that will run during the show. While Susan is on air, the fashion coordinator keeps track of the models' outfits and hands them their clothes when they change outfits. She also puts together the shoes and accessories for each outfit.

"Susan's so friendly and really easy to work with. She likes subtle accessories that don't draw the focus away from the clothes," says Tammy, one of the fashion coordinators who keeps the accessories organized, with a compartmentalized box for earrings and wall pegs for necklaces.

"We've become buds," says Maria, one of the models. "She's always joking around with us."

"Susan comes back to our dressing room after every show to thank us," says Iris. "It means a lot."

"I think she's very down to earth," Sioux adds. "She loves talking to people on air and reading their letters. I'll let you in on a little secret: the hosts don't feel they have to work as hard when Susan's with them on the air. She's just such a natural."

party—no matter how many you throw, you always have a minute of worry that no one will show up! Every week, I'm thrilled when I see the phone light up. It makes me feel great to know people come back week after week.

When the show's over, I head back to the green room and get unhooked from all my cords and microphones. My mother-in-law calls after every show to find out how it went. She and my mother are great coaches. My mother tapes every show—even after all these years she has never missed a show! She lives in Florida, tapes every show and mails the tape to me in New York! Now that's true love. You might think that my day is done now, but this is when I usually meet with buyers, look at samples of upcoming lines, and discuss any issues that may have come up during the show.

My day at QVC usually ends around two or three in the afternoon with a meeting with Terry Heyman. We go over sample garments the manufacturer has made up for us. We check to make sure the colors are right or the pattern is what we wanted. Sometimes we'll see a garment and realize we love a fabric, but it just doesn't look right for that piece (an example is that jacket I told you about earlier). Sometimes we'll realize we have too much blue in a certain grouping, or too many dark colors in general. Then we'll send word back to the manufacturer to change the color of certain items. It takes approximately four weeks from the time we pattern a garment to when we receive the first sample. If we send it back for alterations, it can take another four weeks. It's a long and involved process, but when you see your designs finally brought to life—exactly as you envisioned them—there is nothing in the world like it.

Cleaning Out Your

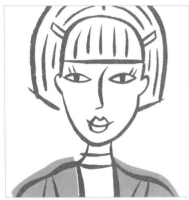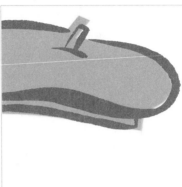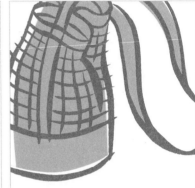

Chapter 2

Closet

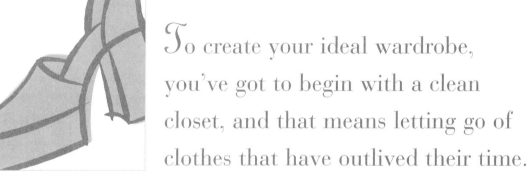

To create your ideal wardrobe, you've got to begin with a clean closet, and that means letting go of clothes that have outlived their time.

What goes in, must come out—the tasseled cowboy shirt from 1993, the prairie skirt from 1983, the toe socks from 1973! They've hung there waiting to come back into style, waiting for you to squeeze back into them, but it's time to face facts. Before you do anything else, you must first weed out all those "some-days" and come to terms with who you are right now—not who you were or who you want to be, but who you are *today*—and be happy to be her.

I know some people think I'm crazy, but I think it's fun to reorganize my closet. I always discover things I'd forgotten about that had slipped behind other pieces or ended up stuffed in the back of a drawer. I take the time to make new combinations from the pieces I have and to evaluate what I might need for the coming season. I try to clean out my closet every six months. I'm fortunate to have plenty of closets in my house, so I keep separate summer and winter closets. I rotate garments into my bedroom

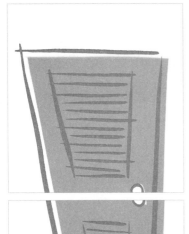

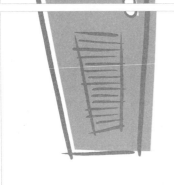

closet with the change of season. Things that I wear all year—my microfiber suits and separates, matte jerseys, or lightweight cardigans—I always keep at hand. But I rotate things like heavy sweaters and shorts when the weather changes. It's important to take stock of your clothes every few months. This way you avoid buying something you already have, and you can quickly gauge what you need to buy.

Parting Is Such Sweet Sorrow

Getting rid of clothing can make you feel guilty. You spent your hard-earned money on something and you feel wasteful tossing it aside after a season or two. All I can say is that if you hung onto everything you bought, you would soon have no room to live. From time to time, you must weed out the closet, and there is no better time to do it than the present. To ease the guilt, start by telling yourself you are going to avoid this pain in the future by shopping primarily for timeless, well-made pieces that will out-last changing trends. Then console yourself by realizing someone else is going to benefit from your newfound organization—you can give clothing you no longer wear to a friend or donate it to someone who needs it.

❋ Friends

When it's time to thin my wardrobe, I make two stacks of what I want to give away. The first stack is for my friends who include girlfriends, relatives, babysitters, and housekeepers—anyone whose personality and sense of style I know. I always put the best pieces in my friends' stack and invite them to sort through it. Make sure you offer clothes appropriate to your friends' tastes; you don't want to accidentally offend a girlfriend, older aunt, or

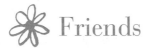

your babysitter. It's always a nice idea to offer your clothes to people close to you first. Once everyone has had her pick, pack up what's left for charity.

Charity Organizations

My second stack (and whatever remains from the friends' stack) goes to charity. These are items that are in good condition but might be out of style or the wrong size. I make sure the clothes are clean and wearable, and I pack them up neatly. There are hundreds of organizations that would love a donation of clothes, from local drama or music schools looking for costumes for their performances, to old standbys like Goodwill or a local charity.

Consignment Shops

If you paid a fortune for something and would like to get a little of the money back, you can always take your clothing to a consignment shop. There is at least one in nearly every large town—they are wonderful sources for prom dresses and bridal-party gowns. They usually list your garment at half of what it originally cost. If they sell it, they phone you and you split the profit.

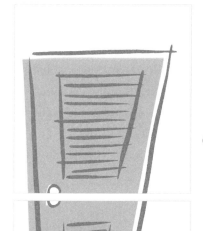

What Needs to Go?

The first thing to go in your quest for your new-look wardrobe is any piece of clothing that doesn't fit. A size-10 dress when you've been a 6 for three years, a slinky skirt that won't pull over your hips, those jeans that you can zip but can't button at the top without cutting off your blood supply, anything that doesn't look great on you. It's hard to let go of clothing you once loved but that no longer fits, especially if the weight loss or gain has been so gradual you've barely noticed. But you've got to do it. Now, I'm

not saying you should toss out every single item that's a little too tight or too baggy. If you are on an exercise regimen and sticking to it, or you are steadily taking off weight, go ahead and keep a few treasured items a size or two too small. But if these treasures make you feel guilty every time you look at them, or if you've been saying to yourself for over a year, "Once I go on that diet, I'll be able to wear that dress again. . ." do yourself a favor and get rid of them. Likewise if you know that you are gaining weight—don't throw away that adorable big shirt. But if your weight has been steady for some time—give away those larger sizes or have them altered to fit your slimmer shape. You need to look good *now*. If you look and feel confident in the present, you'll be able to accomplish a lot more of the goals you set for yourself—including gaining or taking off a few pounds.

 ## Have You Worn It in a Year?

Whether it's because it doesn't really fit, or because you bought it on impulse and it doesn't go with anything else you own, or because your sensibility has changed and it's just not "you" anymore, if you haven't worn an item of clothing for over a year, it's a good sign that you can get rid of it. Weed out ill-fitting and trendy clothes first. If a garment is well made and a classic cut, why not pack it up and look at it again in a year? You might be more in the mood for it then, and it should still be in style. If you look at it a year later and, you still wouldn't wear it, into the give-away pile it goes!

 ## Is It Still in Style?

There is a saying that goes "If you were old enough to wear it once, you're too old to wear it again." We've all watched the seventies creeping back, but most of us who once wore our midriff shirts and hot pants proudly are beyond that now. Even if we still fit into what we wore then, we would probably look silly wearing something designed for a teenager. And somehow the old versions never really look like the new versions they inspire. I recently bought a pair of hip-hugger jeans, but they look a lot fresher and more contemporary than my old Landlubbers ever could! Look at the items in your closet and honestly ask yourself if they are truly still stylish. Lime green spandex has seen its day. It might be time to let go of those neon stirrup pants. How about the shoulder pads on that jacket? Are they subtle, like today's styles, or the linebacker style of the eighties? Things that are blatant examples of old trends need to be weeded from your closet. This also goes for footwear. Because shoes aren't as noticeable, we tend to hang onto them long after the shape of the toe or the height or width of the heel has dated them. Give away shoes that are no longer in style or are worn out, and in the future concentrate on buying classic shoes—and then take very good care of them.

Is the Price Tag Still Attached?

Was it a gift that you didn't have the heart to return? Did you buy it on sale only to get home and find you never wanted to put it on? If the tag is still on a garment after a year, you know what to do with it.

Is It Damaged Beyond Repair?

A lost button on a cardigan is replaceable. Three lost buttons mean a little more work. Stretched buttonholes, frayed cuffs, snags and pills mean a beloved garment needs a fond send-off. Some items of clothing are beyond help. Even donating things that will just have to be thrown away defeats the spirit of charity. If your T-shirts are too stained to wear and bleach doesn't brighten them, or your jeans are not only trendily ripped across the knees but also across the backside, cut them up and use them for rags. Shred old linen shirts and use them in your compost. Natural fibers are sometimes recyclable. Call your local recycling center and find out if they take old clothes.

 ## Do You Love It?

We've come to the final question. There is nothing harder than parting with a truly beloved piece of clothing. A skirt might have taken you on your first date with your husband, or a pair of pants might have gotten you through your first trip to Europe. A young woman I know is so sentimentally attached to two cotton dresses she wore during a summer backpacking in Greece, she can't bear to part with them. They are full of holes, faded by the sun, and no longer fit well, but they remind her of a time when she was happy, independent, and carefree. My advice to her: keep those dresses. They are obviously important to you in the same way a postcard or a souvenir can be. Just don't keep them hanging in your closet, because you are taking up valuable space with something you will never wear. Wrap your dresses in tissue paper and store them as a keepsake with your other travel mementos. No one says you have to get rid of clothing you love. Pack a box of treasures to keep for your children or grandchildren, and store it somewhere dry. Old, colorful clothes are wonderful for playing dress-up, and well-made classic dresses and sweaters will more than likely come back into style.

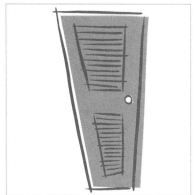

Organization

Every woman has her own method of keeping track of her clothes. What works best for me is to hang *everything* up. I hang my pants together, then my skirts, jackets, and blouses by type. I even hang shells and casual jeans. With everything in one place, I can see it all and make combinations in my head. I like to keep

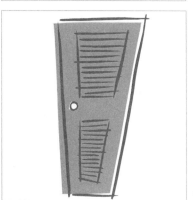

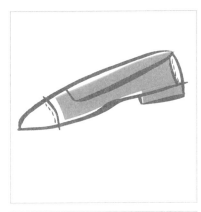

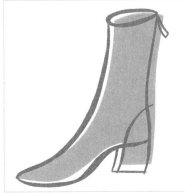

sweaters on shelves so that they are visible. I'll keep tank tops, T-shirts, and underwear in drawers, but that's about it. If I had too much shoved in drawers, I'd forget what I own and wouldn't get the most for my fashion dollar.

You need plenty of good hangers, especially if you are going to hang up everything. Plastic will do, but avoid the wire hangers you get from the dry cleaner. They will stretch the shoulder seams of knits and leave indentations in the fabric. The hangers I like best hang jackets and have clips for a skirt or pants, which let you create outfits by hanging the jacket over a slim skirt or pair of trousers. (If you don't have clipped hangers, hook one around the hook of another). This way you can make up outfits ahead of time and hang them off to the side in their own section.

I clip my pants at the bottom hem or cuff rather than folding them over a hanger or clipping them at the waist. When pants are hung this way, the heavier part hangs down, which keeps the crease crisp and pulls out most wrinkles. It also maximizes space by making them less bulky on the rack. (I don't like to fold pants, because then I have to iron them!) If you have a long dress, you can use a second hanger with clips next to the first hanger and clip the bottom up so it doesn't brush against your shoes or the floor of your closet. Fasten one or two buttons when you hang a blouse so that it doesn't slip off the hanger, and take care when you hang your jackets not to displace their shoulder pads.

When it comes to sweaters, I recommend folding them in half and laying them flat, which makes them wrinkleless. Many times I'll hang up a lighter-weight sweater. At the end of winter, I get all my sweaters dry-cleaned before I put them away for the summer. My dry cleaner returns them folded in great sweater bags that snap closed for easy storage. I fold the bags over a hanger in the winter closet. I've never had trouble with moths if I've had things cleaned before I store them.

I store most of my shoes along the bottom of my closet. I try to color-coordinate them, though I have to confess that about a week after I've straightened up, color groups are once again hopelessly mixed up. I do try to keep them separated by style: one section for dressy shoes, boots in another section, casual and athletic shoes in another section. Because of the business I'm in, I have an extraordinary selection of shoes. I have on-air shoes, off-air shoes, benefit shoes, athletic shoes, comfortable walking and shopping shoes—you name it. If you can afford shoetrees, they really do extend the life of your shoes. They are a bit of a luxury though, and I can't claim to always use them myself.

Now that your closet is straight and you've gotten rid of who you used to be, you can concentrate on who you've become. The second step in creating a confident closet is to take a moment to really think about your likes and dislikes. It's time to decide who you are and what you need from your wardrobe.

Creating Extra Closet Space

If you don't have a spare closet, buy a few large garment boxes and set up a makeshift closet in your attic or finished basement. Places like Hold Everything sell simple garment boxes with built-in hanging racks, as well as fancier, zippered ones. You can also find large plastic storage boxes that will fit under the bed. It's really helpful when organizing your closet to store garments that are simply out of season someplace else—this way you have far fewer things to search through when you're trying to pull together an outfit.

Heels Together!

I recently purchased a fantastic shoe organizer that hangs from the inside of my closet door. Pairs of shoes are stored together in clear plastic compartments. It's easy to see the shoes and it's a great asset to the organization of my closet.

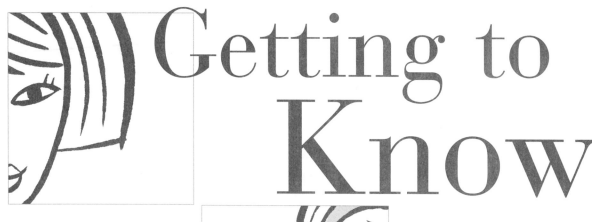

Getting to
Know

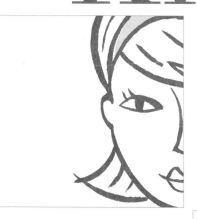

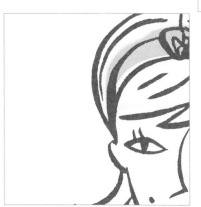

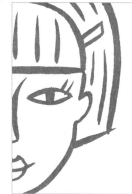

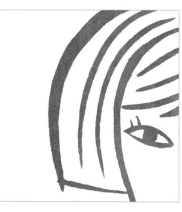

Chapter 3

Yourself

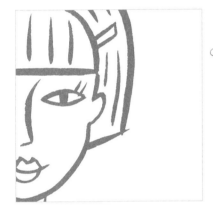

When I was fifteen years old, I went on my very first date. It was with a guy I really liked and he was taking me to the movies. I chose my favorite outfit to look and feel my best.

I had really long hair back then, and I brushed it out. I carefully did my makeup so it would look like I wasn't wearing any. I pulled on my favorite embroidered peasant blouse and faded bell-bottom blue jeans. I thought I looked good and felt great! I went downstairs to model for my mother, and her jaw hit the floor. "You're going out in that?" she gasped. "What's he going to think?"

"He's going to think this is who I am," I answered. "And if he doesn't like the real me, who needs him!"

No one can tell you how to dress. Not your mother, not your boyfriend or husband, not even me. Only you know what makes you feel good. What I want to do in these next few sections is give you some tools to help you identify your likes and dislikes, so that you can avoid buying things you'll never wear and love wearing the things you do buy. Knowing what you like will also help you make the most of your fashion budget.

Knowing What You Like

Have you ever spent a whole lot of money on a piece of clothing, only to find when you got it home that you had nothing at all in your closet to go with it? Maybe it was on sale, maybe it looked really great on the mannequin, or maybe you were just in a hot-pink mood that day. (Of course you have, it was that shirt we just pulled from your closet and gave away—the one with the price tag still attached!) Don't be upset, we all do it from time to time. But that's why it's important to start analyzing your wardrobe and your clothing choices.

People who know fine wine look for certain things in a vintage. They sniff the wine for its aroma, swishing it around to release its bouquet. They look at its color and clarity and taste it for its different subtle flavors. Now, it's certainly okay to sip a wine and say, "This is pretty good," without thinking any more about it, just like it's okay to buy a blouse because you think it's "pretty." But just like a connoisseur of wine looks deeper, so too does a smart shopper. Instead of bouquet, color, and taste, she buys a garment based on color, texture, and silhouette. By judging these three elements, she can decide whether a piece belongs in her wardrobe.

You probably evaluate clothing on these three elements all the time without even thinking about it. When you go out shopping, do you routinely pass by the power suits and make a beeline for the soft velvet dresses? Do you ignore that lovely beige sheath in favor of a bright, bold jumper? Do you touch almost every sweater on the rack before deciding on the one that "just feels right"? You're not alone. Retail stores have done studies that show women are much more tactile than men, and they often choose clothes for their feel. When women shop via a television show or a catalog, they look for clothes that are modeled or have detailed descriptions, so that they can *imagine* how the fabric will feel.

Color

As I mentioned earlier, my background and college major was in art. Most artists work from a palette, or a range of colors that expresses who they are and how they feel. I want you to think for a minute like an artist. Go to your closet. What is your palette? Which colors attract you? I bet if you made stacks of your clothes by color, you'd have one stack that was much higher than all the others. Maybe it's black, because you think black is sophisticated and goes with everything. Maybe your palette is neutral, with a range of soft creams and beiges. Or maybe you own ten red sweaters, two hot pink skirts, and a drawer full of burgundy underwear. It doesn't matter what your palette is— there is no right or wrong one—the point is to identify and work with the range of color that best expresses your personality.

When I look at a color, I don't just examine its tone, I look at its intensity. I break down colors into five intensity groups: Pastels (cool, pale pinks, blues, greens, etc.), mid-tones (vibrant, saturated pastels like deep spring green, melon, deep lavender, etc.), jewel-tones (like emerald green, sapphire, and ruby red), electric brights (lime green, bright orange, neon blue), and warm-tones (chocolate brown, brick red, etc.) Certain colors complement different women's skin and hair tones better than others. I've found that Caucasian women with light hair are washed out by bright colors and shine when they wear pastels and midtones. Asian women, who often have a more yellow cast to their skin, look best in midtones and jewel tones. African American women, and others who have dark complexions, look phenomenal in electric brights and warm tones. They can wear colors that might overpower someone fairer. Once on my TV show, the fashion coordinator put Iris, a stunning black model in a navy blue suit, and dressed Lisa, a fair blonde, in fuchsia. The suit disappeared on Iris and poor Lisa was swallowed up in color. "Switch them! Switch them!" I shouted. Once each was in the outfit that complemented her skin and hair, both women looked fantastic. You need to make sure your palette is working with your complexion and hair color, and not against it.

The color and intensity of your palette can say a lot about you. If you have a lot of navy and chocolate browns, if your racks are full of gray and tan, you are probably a more neutral dresser. You feel most comfortable fitting quietly into social situations, rather than thrusting yourself forward into the limelight. Now this doesn't mean you're a wet rag. On the contrary, many women wear neutral colors so that their personalities don't have to compete with their look. I have a great friend Sandi Sacks, who often wears black and dark colors, which you might think would mean she is a little somber. But in fact, the opposite is true. She has one of the most sparkling personalities of anyone I know. Her subdued clothes are like her backdrop, like the simple velvet lining that shows off a diamond in its case. You wouldn't put a diamond ring in a box lined with paisley—it would get lost! And my friend's bubbly personality shines against the simple colors she chooses.

If you're the sort of woman whose closet is full of bright, vibrant colors, your clothes are probably an extension of your personality, rather than a backdrop to it. You are probably bold, outgoing, and perfectly comfortable in the spotlight. You wear reds and purples and don't shy away from prints and patterns. Putting on a beige suit would make you feel drab and stifled, in the same way another woman might feel clownish in one of your favorite outfits.

So take inventory. Count how many pieces you have in what colors and what intensities. Compare how many prints you have as opposed to solids. Take the time to write down a list of what you have and what color it is. Rank the dominant colors in your wardrobe from one through five, and identify yourself as "Neutral or Bold".

❋ Neutral

Color	Number of pieces	Ranking
Beige		
Black		
Blue		
Brown		
Gray		
Green		
Orange		
Pink		
Purple		
Red		
White		
Yellow		

❋ Bold

Color	Number of pieces	Ranking
Beige		
Black		
Blue		
Brown		
Gray		
Green		
Orange		
Pink		
Purple		
Red		
White		
Yellow		

No Rules

I have no absolute rules for what colors should or should not be worn together. I'm not of the school that says you can't wear white after Labor Day. I think you should wear any color that looks good on you, any time of year. I also think the idea of colors "clashing" is a little outdated. As long as you choose colors that share the same basic intensity, it's hard to go wrong. I used to think that colors like purple and red clashed—but even that combination can look stunning, as long as it complements your coloring. But you could easily misstep if you wore an electric bright or warm tone with a jewel tone. You also want to be careful with prints. While you can wear two prints together if one is large and the other is small and subtle, two bold prints together almost always spell disaster.

Texture

Okay, go back to your closet. I want you to touch every single thing hanging there. Open your drawers and caress your clothes. Go ahead, nobody's looking! You are trying to get a sense of the overall texture of your wardrobe. You are feeling for the general crispness or fluidity, the stiffness or softness of the clothes you own. Which pieces feel best to you? Which pieces feel too stiff, or maybe too flimsy? A fabric's texture is sometimes called its "hand". So when I say a certain fabric has a soft hand or a

Color	Number of pieces	Ranking
Beige		
Black		
Blue		
Brown		
Gray		
Green		
Orange		
Pink		
Purple		
Red		
White		
Yellow		

✳ Fluid

Color	Number of pieces	Ranking
Beige		
Black		
Blue		
Brown		
Gray		
Green		
Orange		
Pink		
Purple		
Red		
White		
Yellow		

brushed hand, I'm speaking of the general feel of the fabric.

Do you own several thick wool jackets? Are there racks of flannel and gabardine pants? Is that a neat linen vest peeking out? You are probably a woman who prefers structured fabrics, fabrics that look crisp and keep their shape.

If instead you have a closet full of silky, lighter-weight clothes, such as swingy long skirts and unstructured jackets, you probably prefer fluid fabrics. You gravitate toward velvet pants and soft silk blouses instead of creased wool and starched cotton. Just like knowing your palette, to build a strong wardrobe, you need to know what kind of textures make you feel great. Take inventory, and based on how many pieces in your closet fall into either category, identify yourself as "Structured" or "Fluid".

The Fabric Revolution

There has been a revolution in textiles over the past few years, and women on a budget are the first to benefit. With the advent of microfibers, (extremely thin polyester threads) fabric can be woven much tighter, giving it a soft hand that polyester never had before. I'm sure you remember that stiff, flat, cheesy-feeling cloth from the seventies that just screamed, "I'm cheap!" Now, with the new microfibers, you can't tell if a garment is real silk or synthetic, 100 percent wool or poly-wool. Not only are these new materials less expensive, best of all, they are also fully washable. No more dry cleaning bills! I love microfibers! This textile revolution has allowed me to offer my customers a huge range of fabrics—at very affordable prices.

Silhouette

Is your closet full of tailored, carefully fitted pieces? Do you have racks of straight skirts and crisp cotton blouses? For your active wear, do you reach for a pair of pleated linen walking shorts and an oxford-cloth shirt? If so, you probably love timeless classics that never go out of style.

If on the other hand, you look into your closet and see a pair of magenta hot pants, a fringed leather vest, a plaid jacket, and a lacy little sheath, you might be of the more dramatic bent. Personally, I'm drawn to both classics and drama. Hanging in my closet next to several classic suits, I have a pair of faux leather pants (faux leather, or fake leather, is much cheaper than real leather) and an orange, sleeveless, chunky, knit sweater that I adore. Now, this is not a practical piece— if it's cold out you need some sleeves and when it's warm enough to go sleeveless, it's too hot for a chunky knit! Most of what I design are simple, easy-to-wear pieces. I focus on classic styles—nothing too kooky, nothing too severe, and nothing that you need the perfect figure to wear. But because I am a little dramatic too, I like to add something fun to even my most traditional designs.

Take a good look at the silhouette and general style of your clothes. Are you more "Traditional," more "Dramatic," or even a little of both?

Your Personal Style Profile

So are you Neutral Structured Traditional? Or Bold Fluid Dramatic? Maybe you're Bold Structured Traditional or Neutral Fluid Dramatic or you may be Neutral Structured for work, but Bold Fluid at home.

You can be any combination at all and still be a fantastic dresser. What's important is that you keep who *you* are in mind when you add a new piece to your wardrobe. If your closet is full of cream and brown, you might want to buy that sweater in pale pink rather than vivid turquoise. And vice versa, if you're all about bright prints and crinkled crepe, that pair of navy flannel trousers is going to get awfully lonely in your closet. I am not saying you shouldn't have one or two startling pieces in your wardrobe. I know a very fashionable young woman, a Neutral Structured Traditional, who recently purchased a hot pink, embroidered mini-dress. Does the color go with anything else in her wardrobe? No. But interestingly enough, it's a carefully fitted garment, made of a heavier raw silk. In cut and texture, her minidress actually fits in with other pieces she likes and owns. Even when buying a bold piece, she stuck to two of the key elements of her personal style profile, and she loves having a color that's out of her natural palette to make her feel extra fabulous on those very special occasions.

Is Less More?

"Is it better to save your money for a few good pieces, or buy cheaper, up-to-the-minute clothes and have more to choose from?" Over and over I'm asked this question, and I wish I could give you a definite answer. In the end, I think it boils down to how you have identified yourself. If you like well-tailored, structured clothes in timeless colors, you might want to save and buy a handful of expensive garments, making sure that they coordinate perfectly. If, on the other hand, you've identified yourself as a bold, dramatic sort, you probably couldn't keep yourself from buying trendy clothes if you tried. When I was younger, I tried to be sensible and tell myself I'd choose only a few good pieces. I diligently saved for one traditional suit, but then the rest of my money went to peasant blouses and bell-bottom trousers and jeans! Now that I'm older, I tend to make more of an investment. I have a tan suit with pants that I've worn for the past six years. I have another great suit in black. One set of trousers has a narrower leg, the other has a wider one. I wear them a whole lot more than I wear my orange, chunky sweater and faux leather pants.

The best news is that with new, washable synthetics, even the most classic look won't cost you a fortune. You can buy a fully lined poly-wool suit for a fraction of what the same natural-fiber outfit would cost you. And today's beautiful microfiber blouses add a new and exciting look to simple classic suits.

Body Shapes

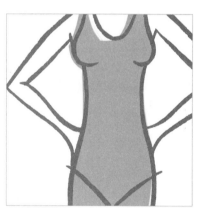

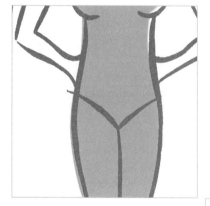

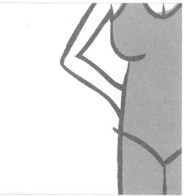

Chapter 4

We all look in the mirror a hundred times a day. We brush our hair, apply our makeup, check to see that our hems haven't fallen in the back and that our hose haven't run. But how often do we really see ourselves?

I mean from the top of our scalps to the polish on our toenails? I would bet that you haven't given your entire body any serious scrutiny since you were a teenager, except maybe to sigh and say, "I sure look fat today," or "Why don't I fill out this blouse?" It's easy—far too easy—to criticize. It's much harder to evaluate ourselves honestly, to assess our flaws and admire our assets. Our bodies are always changing. We're gaining or losing weight, we're firming up or we're starting to sag. A lot of fashion mistakes are made because we refuse to look in the mirror and see what's before us today. Very few of us have been born with perfect bodies. We all need to get a realistic sense of our good and our less-good features so that we can learn little tricks to help out Mother Nature. To do that, we must identify and understand our body types.

Mirror, Mirror on the Wall

Your new look starts with confronting that full-length mirror on the inside door and taking a level, loving look at your body. To take this exercise seriously, set aside a time when you won't be interrupted by anyone or anything. If you have a best friend who you trust enough to let her see you half-naked, invite her over to help you take measurements. Then you do the same for her. I know some people will tell you to stand nude in front of the mirror and take a good look, but I say, "no way!" If I were standing nude, I know I'd get distracted by that little bulge here or that little dimple there, and I'd start beating myself up about not exercising regularly. Also, if you're older, certain things will sag if you're naked that don't when you wear your normal foundation garments. I'd say put on the kind of bra and panties you usually wear, and over those some black leggings and a close-fitting tank top. You want to show off your form while making sure you're supported. Using your waist as a starting point, take a washable marker or soft makeup pencil or lip-liner and draw your outline on the mirror. Now stand back.

What do you see? Are you heavier on the bottom? On the top? Sometimes it takes something as impartial as an outline to show you your real shape. You might be convinced you have thunder thighs, but when you examine your drawing, you may find you're far more in proportion than you thought.

Next we need to get even more scientific. To get a really accurate picture of your body shape, you need to take measurements, see page 133. This is when it's really handy to have a friend to help you. Whatever you do, don't focus on your weight—we'll discuss sizes later. For the purposes of this chapter, you can be petite or full-figured. It's not weight that matters in identifying your body shape, it's proportion. I have names for the basic body types: "Hourglass", "Fan", "Bell", "Full Moon", and "Bamboo." You might ask how I came up with these names. I have a beautiful Oriental screen in my living room, painted with ladies whose poses suggested these shapes to me!

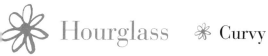 Hourglass

* Curvy
* Breasts and hips in basically equal proportion
* Tapered waist

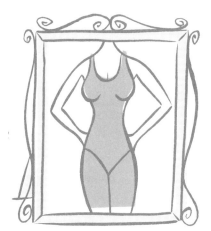

Lucky you! You can wear just about anything. You simply need to recognize your good fortune and not cover yourself up. I have a neighbor who has a marvelous figure, but she doesn't know how to optimize it. She wears dowdy tunic tops and leggings, which do nothing to show off her shape. My advice to Hourglass women: if you've got it, flaunt it! Wear those form-fitting tops and shapely short skirts. Just be careful when it comes to your height. If you are a short Hourglass, don't wear jackets and skirts that are too long and will swallow you up. The same goes for short jackets and skirts if you are especially tall. (We'll discuss length and hemline more in the section The Perfect Fit. See page 58.)

What to Buy

Skirt: Short and long skirts look equally great on you. Try a sarong or an A-line. If you are very curvy, you might want to steer clear of pencil skirts or long, tightly fitted straight skirts. Trousers: Classic straight-legged trousers look best. Bell-bottoms or other pants with a slight flare that mirror your curves can be fun.

Jacket: You probably look best in a fitted jacket with a little flaring peplum that lies nicely over your hips, but you can get away with a tailored tuxedo jacket or even a mandarin bolero jacket.

Dress: An A-line would suit you perfectly, but you can experiment with spaghetti straps or a halter.

Bathing Suit: Why not try a bikini?

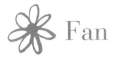 # Fan

* Top heavy

* Wide shoulders

* Narrow hips

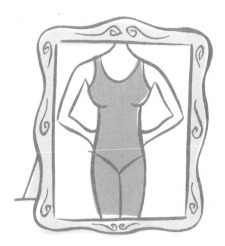

You are shaped more like an inverted triangle with broad shoulders that taper down to narrow hips and fantastic legs. Your legs are your best feature and the trick is to showcase them while softening your more squarish shoulders. The most important thing for Fan women to remember is to keep things simple on the top. Avoid shoulder pads at all costs, and don't wear shirts with large prints that will call attention to your upper body. It's also good to avoid white on top. Use this as a rule of thumb: darker colors minimize, lighter colors accentuate. You want to draw the eye down, not up. Throw away the chokers and short chunky beads. A long necklace will work wonders on you.

What to Buy

Skirt: Choose a short slim skirt to show off those great legs. You can also wear a longer slim skirt, or a pencil, but stay away from things that flair. You might think a tulip or trumpet skirt will even you out top-to-bottom, but it will just make you look square.

Trousers: Choose narrow-legged trousers rather than wide-legged pants, which can make you look chunky.

Jacket: Choose a jacket with an open neckline, like a fitted tuxedo jacket. Anything with a V-neck will make your upper body look less broad. It's best to avoid high necklines like mandarin or grandfather collars because they bring the eye up to your wide shoulders, your least flattering feature.

Dress: Avoid halter dresses or dresses with puff sleeves. These will make you look like a linebacker. Aim instead for V- or scoop-neck dresses in dark colors. Bell sleeves with a flare around the wrist are good; they will draw attention away from your upper body.

Bathing Suit: Go for a lower neck line with a criss-cross front. Show off your legs with a suit cut higher on the sides.

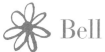

Bell

* Bottom heavy

* Wide hips

* Narrow shoulders

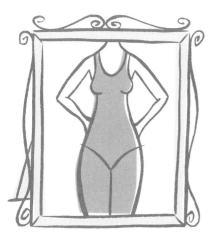

You are the opposite of the Fan. Your shoulders are narrow or sloping; you often have a smaller torso and bust; and most of your weight is carried below the hips. (One piece of good news: if you have to carry any extra weight, it is healthier to carry it around the hips and thighs. It puts you at less of a risk for heart trouble and for some diseases like diabetes.)

Your upper body is your best feature, and we want to show it off, while minimizing your wider hips. You are a perfect candidate for shoulder pads. They will draw the eye up and create a more balanced shape. You want to wear darker colors on the bottom and lighter colors up top, again to pull focus toward your chest. Chunky knit sweaters with straight-legged jeans are a great combination for you. Stay away from textured fabrics below the belt, which will only make your bottom look bulkier.

What to Buy

Skirt: An A-line is definitely the way to go. It falls gracefully from the hips and hides any extra bulge in the thigh area. Look for loose, flowing fabrics that won't cling. Don't get anything that's too tight. For skirts and trousers alike, avoid pleats and go for a flat-front.

Trousers: Straight-legged pants such as stovepipe trousers will make you look taller and slimmer, but you'll look like you fill up wide-legged pants, even if you're not that heavy. You should steer away from trousers that have bulky elastic waists and belts that call attention to your midsection. Reach instead for flat-front trousers with elastic in the back only.

Jacket: Your hips will seem to flare out below a short jacket, which will make you appear even smaller on top. You should choose a jacket that falls below the hip, or even a bit longer, to cover your upper thighs and rear. A duster with a high side-slit will give you the coverage of a long jacket, and can really spice up your wardrobe.

Dress: Choose an A-line with shoulder pads. Most necklines will work well on you, especially boatnecks, V-necks, and collared necklines.

Bathing Suit: Bell-shaped women tend to want to cover up below, which is a good idea. Sarongs work great as cover-ups, but the bathing suit itself should not have longer legs or short little skirts. Little skirts call attention to wide hips. Instead, reach for a bathing suit with high-cut legs that will make your legs look longer and your hips less wide. If you have a good stomach, you can also wear a twopiece suit or bikini. The break in the suit will draw the eye up and away from a heavier bottom.

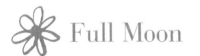 Full Moon ❋ Rounded or square torso

❋ Straight waist, untapering.

❋ Thin legs

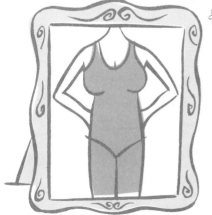

You have a rounded or square upper body and thin, shapely legs. You may find it hard to dress because too often clothes cut you across the middle, drawing attention to a thicker waistline. Luckily, your legs are to die for. It's really a matter of showing off your legs, much as it is for a Fan. I once saw a woman in a coffee shop who was a Full–Moon—she was incredibly stylish. She

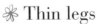

wore a blouson top (a billowy tunic-style shirt with elastic at the bottom) that came in at the hips and had a mandarin collar. She completed the outfit with a pair of skintight leggings that showed off her best feature. It was the perfect outfit because it hid her lack of a waistline and called attention to her long, slender legs.

What to Buy

Skirt: A flat-front slim skirt with an elastic waist at the back would probably be the most comfortable and flattering. Stay away from dirndl skirts and anything that binds at the waist.
Trousers: Long, straight-legged trousers, with a flat-front and elastic back, will compensate for your larger waistline, while still tapering over your slender legs. Avoid anything with a belt.
Jacket: Always choose a longer, loose tunic-jacket that falls below the hip and backside. You want to avoid anything fitted that tapers at the waist. Dolman and bell sleeves look especially flattering on you.
Dress: Try a shorter A-line dress that begins to flare under the bustline and not at the waist. A blouson dress that blouses over the torso then tapers at the hips would also be lovely.
Bathing Suit: A one-piece suit with a little skirt will make you look perfectly in proportion.

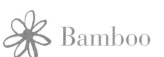 Bamboo

 Tall and thin

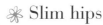 Slim hips

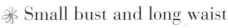 Small bust and long waist

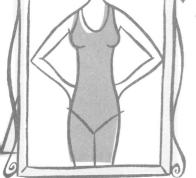

Congratulations! Your body shape is very popular today and you can wear almost anything with confidence. Not all tall, thin women grow up feeling like supermodels, however. Many have been made to feel self-conscious about their height and some have had difficulty finding clothes that fit. Luckily, along with stores that cater to plus-size women, many shops carry a line of clothing for taller women.   As for jewelry, a long necklace will make you look taller, a choker of chunky pearls or a scarf around the neck will make your upper torso look fuller. If you want to minimize your Bamboo shape, don't dress all in one color. Wear a light shirt and dark pants and add a belt to divide your length.

What to Buy

Skirt: You can wear just about any shape, from a dirndl to a pencil. Skirts that fall just above or just below the knee will minimize rather than accentuate your height.

Trousers: Cuffed pants look great on taller women. You can also get away with wide-legged pants that fall from the hips. You might want to steer away from leggings and stovepipe pants that could make your legs look sticklike.

Jacket: You want to work with the lean lines of your body by choosing a longer tailored jacket that falls just below the hips. Avoid jackets with peplums that flare at the hips you don't have.

Dress: You look great in a turtleneck dress or in a long straight sheath. Really, you have the type of body that can wear almost anything. Experiment!

Bathing Suit: Don't buy a suit cut too high in the legs, it will make you look even taller. Color-blocked and print suits will look great on you.

The Perfect Fit

I can't tell you how many times I've seen a woman in a gorgeous, expensive outfit that looked awful on her, simply because it didn't fit properly. A blouse was too tight across the chest or sagged in the back; trousers showed panty lines or bunched at the ankle. She might have spent a fortune, but she looked terrible—which means that she ended up making a poor investment. A good fit is absolutely essential. Knowing how to buy clothes that really fit you is just as important as knowing your body type.

Every designer uses different names for different sizes. A "small" for one designer might be a size 6, while for another, it could be a 4. It's maddening to try on a size 8—which you've always worn—and find you can barely squeeze into it. Don't despair and assume you've gained weight. Sizes are dependent on the cut of a garment and they can vary wildly from designer to designer.

I try to stick to a simple standard. I design "small" to be a 6 to 8; "medium" 10 to 12; "large" 14 to 16. I'll sometimes design an "X-large", which is size 18 to 20. These are called Misses sizes. I also design for plus-size women, in sizes "1X" (22 to 24), "2X" (26 to 28), and "3X" (30 to 32). I offer petites in a few items. My petite sizes range from small through 3X. Petite women are not necessarily tiny women, they are merely proportionately shorter. If a woman is four feet, eleven inches tall and wears a 1X, a petite 1X would fit her best because the regular 1X size may be too long in many places.

Knowing your size is important, but you won't really know if a garment fits until you try it on. Too often, women who are feeling a little overweight buy a size too big, thinking they can hide those little bulges inside loose clothes. This is always a mistake. If your clothes are too big, people will assume that you are filling them up underneath. On the other hand, you want to avoid the opposite pitfall of "tight equals sexy." Unless you have a perfect body, a shirt or skirt that is skintight will make you look heavier. Supertight clothes show off every dimple and bulge and tend to look cheap. What you want is a happy medium—clothes that show off the outline of your body, without either hiding it or revealing too much.

How To Tell If Your Clothes Fit?

The "Hug Test" is one quick way to tell if any top or jacket fits. Stand in front of a mirror and hug yourself as tightly as possible. Are your arms constricted? Does it tug so much across the back that you can't bring your arms around to touch your back? Next lift your arms high in the air. Do you have complete range of motion? Does the shirttail come out of your waistband and ride up your stomach? Now put your hands behind your back. Is there a gap between the second and third buttons across your bustline? If you answered yes to any of these questions, your shirt or jacket is too small. Now look in the mirror and see if it is sagging anywhere. Is there too much fabric under your bustline? Does it bunch up below your shoulder blades in the back? Does the hem of the shirt hit you far below the midpoint of your hip? If so, the garment you've picked out is too big. You want your shirts and jackets to fit closely without bunching or stretching. But remember that different styles and different fabrics will have different fits. For example, a structured wool jacket might not give you the ease of motion that its peachskin counterpart would, but it still shouldn't feel excessively binding. If it does, it doesn't fit.

For trousers and skirts, you can try a variation of the Hug Test that I call the "Squat Test." Put on a garment and do a deep knee bend. Could someone standing behind you see all the way down a gap at the back waistband? Does the fabric pull across your buttocks or cut into your crotch? Do your knees feel like they are pushing through the fabric? Now stand up and bend forward. Does the waistband cut painfully into your stomach? Does the hem of the skirt or the pants ride up? If you're wearing pants, hold onto a chair and swing your leg forward and backward to see if you have ample range of motion. If you are trying on a skirt, sit down and see if the skirt has enough room in the seat or if it rides up too far. If you have access to steps, make sure your skirt is not too tight to climb them.

Things To Look For in a...

Jacket

A good jacket completes a classic look, so it's very important it fit impeccably. Do the Hug Test to see if you have gaping buttons; there is nothing less flattering than a jacket that is too snug across the bust. Feel down the bodice to make sure you cannot gather up too much loose fabric. The jacket should be snug but not constricting. (You certainly don't want a jacket so tight—or in a material so thin—that you can see rolls of flesh underneath!) If the jacket has side or back vents, make sure they lie flat and don't gap. The collar should also lie flat in the back and not stand up or fall away from the nape of your neck. Choose a style that hits you at a flattering length. If you are long waisted, a short-waisted jacket will not look good on you. And vice versa, if you are shorter, you'll be swallowed up in a jacket that hits below your hips.

Blouse

A blouse should fit very similarly to a jacket, but you have more leeway in the tightness category. There are many flattering form-fitted tops, but make sure they don't pull at the critical points of the bustline, under the bust, and at the shoulders. A top should never be so tight that bra straps or rolls are visible. The shoulder seam should not fall too far below the apex of the shoulder. Pay careful attention to the fit at the neckline. If you are wearing a high collar, make sure it's not so loose that it sags in the front, or so tight that you look like you're choking.

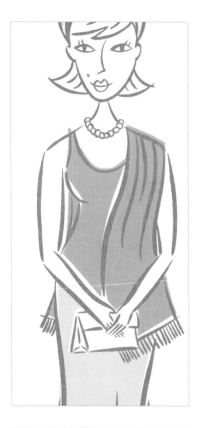

Dress

It is much easier to find a dress that fits well. A classic A-line is flattering on everyone and should fall in a loose triangle from about the center of the ribcage. Be careful of the hemline. If you are short, don't buy a floor-length dress unless you are prepared to wear some very high platform shoes with it. On the other hand, if you are tall, a dress that hits you two-thirds of the way down your thigh will appear skimpy. Beware of clingy dresses unless you have a stunning figure. A dress should never hug you so tightly that your panty lines are showing.

Trousers

More than any other piece of clothing, it is critical that trousers fit well. The rise (the distance from waist to crotch) has to be perfect, not too long and not too short. The rear of a pair of pants is very important; if they are not well fitted, they will make your backside look out of shape. The thigh area has to fit perfectly, not too tight, but not too wide. You never want the fabric to look like it's straining across the thigh because it will make you appear heavy. To some degree, the fit across the thigh also depends on the fabric. Lycra and denim can fit a little closer than gabardine or wool. Silk and peachskin call for a more draped fit. As for length, in a classic trouser the hem or the bottom of the cuff should just brush the top of your foot—you don't want either bunched-up fabric or too much sock showing. Try on trousers in the shoes you'll most often wear with them. And remember, you can always shorten a pair of pants, but if you buy them too short, there is nothing you can do. Since the fit of a pair of trousers is critical, you may have to try twenty different styles to find one that fits really well. When you find that perfect fit, I recommend looking for that same designer when buying your next pair.

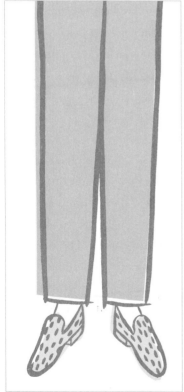

Is It Well Made?

Besides making sure your clothes fit, you want to make certain they are well made. After all, you are spending your hard-earned money, and you want the satisfaction of knowing the designer and manufacturer have paid attention to detail. There are certain things to look for to determine if a garment is well made:

❋ Most button-front shirts should have workable buttons and vent openings in the cuffs in case you want to roll up your sleeves. I also like to see a cuff with a pleat, which helps the drape.

❋ Look inside your jacket. If it is not lined, the seam edges should have serging (a tight stitch to keep the fabric from unraveling). Serged edges prevent fraying, although it is much cheaper to produce a jacket without them.

❋ Make sure the seams are straight and well pressed. A garment that has been made too quickly will not be well made.

❋ Make sure the seams are sewn tightly and evenly. Sometimes manufacturers cut corners by not stopping production and taking the time to change the tension on the sewing machines when necessary. They'll do an order of woven trousers and then an order of jersey trousers. These two fabrics call for different tensions and threads, and better manufacturers will change threads and adjust the machines accordingly. Look at the number of stitches per inch; you can pull the seam tight and count them. There should be between ten and twelve stitches per inch. If there are six or seven, the garment is of lesser quality.

❋ Make sure print patterns match up at the seams. This is especially important with plaids. The patterns of cheaply made garments will not match up.

❋ Look at the buttonholes to make sure that they are well finished and that there are no loose threads. Loose threads on a garment are often a giveaway. At the factory, manufacturers are supposed to "clean" the garment, in other words, to snip the loose threads. If they are rushing an order, they sometimes won't take the time. Use your judgment. If you see a loose thread but the garment looks to be well made overall, they probably just missed a thread. If the garment seems cheaply made, you can bet it is.

❋ Check for pilling. Jersey knits, fleeces, and acrylics will inevitably pill, but you don't want to buy something that is already showing signs of pilling before you've even worn it. I did a polar-fleece jacket and even though it cost extra money, I put an antipill finish on it. It greatly increased the life span of the jacket.

Building Your Wardrobe

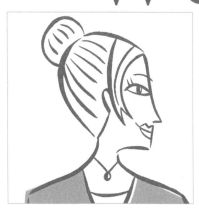

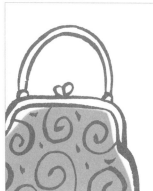

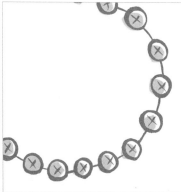

Chapter 5

On the air, I often talk about the five anchors of any woman's wardrobe—the pieces around which all her other clothes will pivot.

I can't stress the importance of these garments enough. They will take you to the office and out to dinner. They will be the clothes you reach for nearly every day to mix and match and dress up with accessories. They should be the most carefully chosen pieces in your closet and as versatile as possible.

What fabric you choose for these pieces will depend on how you've identified yourself in Chapter Three. If you prefer Structured textures, buy your anchor pieces in wool or gabardine; if you are more comfortable in Fluids, you might buy them in peachskin or matte jersey. Make sure that whatever the fabric, these garments are well made and will hold up. You want to get as much wear out of your staples as possible; they should last you years and years if you take good care of them. The fabric is up to you, but even if you are the most dramatic of women, I urge you to choose neutral, classic colors for these five pieces. Please don't buy a three hundred-dollar jacket in this season's hottest color, even if you absolutely love it, until you have these five pieces in one of the neutral colors: black, chocolate brown, gray, camel, or navy. I also want to debunk the myth that you should

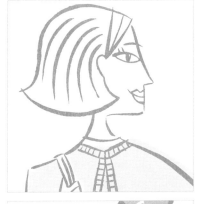

spend a lot on a special-occasion dress, such as an evening gown, only to skimp on everyday wear because it is less "special." If you are going to wear a garment every week, it will pay for itself much sooner than that one-time gown will.

Five Easy Pieces

Let's pretend for a minute that your closet is completely empty, nothing but hangers and space, and you have five hundred dollars to spend. With that, you can easily buy the five anchors of your wardrobe.

I would spend:

❋ Two hundred dollars on a really good jacket. You want to be able to wear it all year, so don't choose a heavy wool or a light silk. I would pick a fully lined, well-made gabardine that is seasonless. Black is a good choice because it's both versatile and sophisticated. If you think black is too severe, go for navy or a deep gray or a warm brown. Try to get true colors, or you may have difficulty matching your staples to your shoes and handbags.

❋ Seventy-five dollars on a pair of classic trousers. If you are tall, they can be smartly cuffed, if you are shorter, like me, you'll probably want to go for a simple, well-stitched hem. I would pick a pair of flat-front, straight-legged trousers—not too tight, not too full—that just hit the top of the heel of your favorite shoes. If not already part of a suit, make sure you buy your trousers in the same shade as your jacket.

❋ Fifty dollars on a slim skirt. I think a slim skirt is usually a better choice than an A-line or a full skirt, because for business situations it is the most classic and conservative. Buy a slim skirt that hits just at the knee or a few inches above. You don't want a miniskirt, no matter what you see on television. Like the trousers, if the skirt is not already a part of a suit, make sure you buy it in the same color as the jacket.

❋ Fifty dollars on a white or ivory blouse with a button front and classic cuffs. This blouse will go with everything you own. You can pair it with your trousers one day, with your slim skirt the next. I would try to buy a blouse with lapels that mirror your jacket's lapels. Choose a notched blouse collar for a jacket with notched lapels, or a shawl-collared blouse for a shawl-collared jacket. This way, if you want to wear your blouse collar on the outside of your jacket, it won't distract from the lines of the jacket. A soft microfiber or crisp cotton is a good choice for this blouse. If you prefer cotton, try one that has been woven with a small amount of Lycra, which makes a blouse more form-fitting and feminine. Although three-quarter-length sleeves are very fashionable right now, I'd still go for a traditional sleeve for your staple blouse.

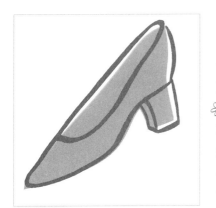

❋ Fifty dollars on a short-sleeved shell with a jewel neckline. This should also be a neutral color, but choose something different from the classic white. For your shell, try a soft blue or pink or an ivory in either a microfiber or thin cashmere. You'll wear it under your jacket, with your skirt, and with your trousers. You'll be able to pair it with almost anything new you buy.

❋ The remaining seventy-five dollars is for a pair of medium-heeled leather shoes that you can wear with your anchor garments. Get them in basic black to go with any of the darker colors and you'll always have shoes to wear, no matter what outfit you put together. And medium heels are most often appropriate.

These five easy pieces will get you through almost any social situation you can imagine. Let's lay out an imaginary week at the office:

❋ Day one: jacket, white blouse, slim skirt

❋ Day two: shell and trousers

❋ Day three: jacket, shell, slim skirt

✳ Day four: white blouse and trousers

✳ Day five: shell and slim skirt

Best of all, any of these looks can be dressed up to carry you through the evening. If you come into work in a shell, jacket, and slim skirt with medium heels, simply remove the jacket, exchange the classic shoes for something strappier, and clasp on some chunky pearls or a long necklace. You're ready to go out to dinner or an evening event.

For my fashion line, I design between ten and twelve "groups" each Winter and Summer season. Within each group, I might design a sweater, a long duster vest, a pair of novelty stylish trousers. But the core of each group, the garments no wardrobe can be without, are definitely the five anchor pieces. I'll always include two pairs of trousers, two skirts (usually a knee-length and a long), two jackets, two blouses, and two shells. You see, it doesn't make any sense for me to design a great vest, if I don't already have the pieces to layer under it. Without a slim skirt or a pair of trousers to match with a duster, there is no point in making it. I'll use twenty different prints per season, but I'll always pair them in some combination with my solid anchor pieces. Your five anchor pieces are indispensable. When you think of them as the core of any fashion grouping, you are shopping like a designer designs!

Today's Little Black Dress

You might think it would have become a cliché by now, but we must take a minute to discuss the Little Black Dress. I've been asked, "Is black passé? Can we now talk about the Little Red Dress or the Little Pink Dress?" My answer, "No." Black can never be passé. It will never go out of style or be anything other than sophisticated and elegant.

You can never go wrong if you have a simple black dress in your closet. In fact, once you have your anchor pieces, think about getting a classic black sheath. It will do so much for your wardrobe, you could even call it your "Sixth Easy Piece." Like your Five Easy Pieces, your black sheath will take you so many places—to the office or dressed up to an elegant affair.

When I was young, my ideal Little Black Dress was a flirty, flippy little thing, short with skimpy spaghetti straps. As I've gotten older, I've grown a bit more sophisticated. Now when I talk of my Little Black Dress, it's a classic sheath that I wear more seriously. This sheath takes me everywhere. I wear it so many different ways. I'll wear it under a jacket, or I'll dress it up with a pair of chunky pearl earrings. I'll wear it over a white Lycra-knit T-shirt and pair it with suede boots. I'll put a belt with it. Recently, I bought a jacket with a removable fur collar that's the same length as the dress. Now I have a super jacket-and-dress ensemble. And I can wear the jacket with a long gown or take the collar off and wear it over a pair of classic trousers.

If I am going to an event in the fashion industry and pink is the color of the season—and I want everyone to know I know pink is the color—I might buy a Little Pink Dress, but I'll only wear it once or twice. It won't become my all-time favorite dress and because it is trendy, I may tire of it when pink is out of style next year. I probably would have been a whole lot smarter if I had said, "I won't be a follower and I love the classic look of black. And that's what I'm going to wear." But like anyone else, I get excited and want to wear the newest fashion color of the season. Okay, end of lecture.

Accessorizing With Clothing

I've said it over and over on TV, and I'll say it again here: if you only have a certain amount of money to spend, spend more on your clothes than on your accessories. Once you have established your basic wardrobe, changing your jewelry wardrobe is a great way to give your basic look a new twist and it can cost much less than changing your entire wardrobe of clothing. I think that

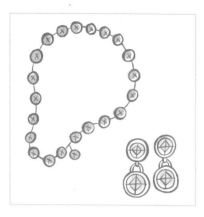

clothing can create a bigger impact than jewelry just because it is more visible. But the small touches are important too. Although people first look at the overall you--the big picture, as they spend more time with you and are sitting next to you, they pick up on the details. I would personally much rather spend forty dollars on a really great vest than on a ring that doesn't really change the big picture look of an outfit. But I do love to buy jewelry and especially watching QVC, I am always seeing a ring or a pair of earrings that I just have to have.

I'm not saying this because I design clothes for a living. It just makes common sense. If you want to jazz up your classic anchor pieces, buy a shirt in the season's "in" color. You can wear it instead of your ivory shell and completely change your look. Or get a duster vest in a great print—it will do more for you than that little pair of earrings. For a more classic look, try a cashmere sweater draped over the shoulders to add color to your classic suit. The next week you can wear the same sweater under your jacket. If you have to stick to a budget, be smart about your extras. Buy items that do double duty. When I buy accessories, I'd rather spend money on a great new handbag to coordinate with my shoes rather than a bracelet that doesn't make a statement. Of course I love jewelry, but those pieces are extras after my wardrobe is complete.

Coats

You wear a coat to keep you warm, but why not also think of it as a fashion accessory? A great coat can completely change the look of your outfit. I love coats, and I probably have too many of them—if that's possible! I have everything from a fun faux fur to a conservative trench coat. I've just designed a great reversible jacket that is solid on one side and quilted on the other. But as with other extras; you need to make sure you have the basics before you indulge your imagination—and empty your bank account!

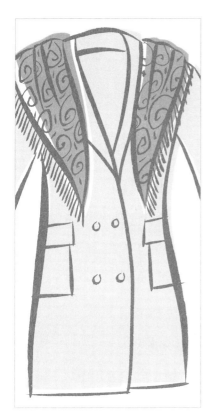

First and foremost, you need one black wool coat. If your palette is navy or brown or gray, you can opt for one of those colors, though black is the safest because it goes with absolutely everything. Choose a coat with a basic button front and a hemline that falls midcalf or below. You might want to look for one with a removable collar and cuffs which gives you two looks in one coat. This will be your everywhere coat. It goes with a long dress or a sweater and jeans. It takes you out to dinner or on vacation. Don't skimp—make sure the fabric is top quality and the coat well made. This is a great item to buy at an off-price store or outlet mall because it should not follow this minute's trends. Your basic wool coat should be classic enough to last you many years.

Once you've got your black wool coat, you can expand as your budget allows. I would say the next item on the list should be a hip-length or mid-thigh A-line swing coat; look for something reversible. A suede or leather jacket is also a great addition. If you live anywhere with seriously cold weather, a long down coat is a must. Unless you are skinny, make sure the quilting is stitched flat, or you'll end up looking like the Michelin Tire man! You should also consider investing in a nice raincoat with a removable lining that can do double duty in winter and summer.

On special occasions you may want to trade your coat for a shawl or wrap made from cashmere, sheep's wool, silk, or microfiber. If you choose the less expensive varieties, you can get a colorful array to go with your dressier clothes or evening wear. While it's true that coats are fashion items, they are first and foremost protection against the weather. Make sure your coat can do its duty. This is not the time to sacrifice function for fashion.

$\mathcal{F}$abrics for Winter and Summer

When choosing your wardrobe, be aware of your garments' seasonableness. Below is a list of summer and winter fabrics. I've also broken them down into Structured and Fluid.

Some fabrics like silk, peachskin, and matte jersey can be worn all year long. Angora and velvet might look a little strange in the summer, but designers are experimenting and adding little touches here and there even in

Summer

Structured	Fluid
Canvas	Cotton/acrylic
Chambray	Cotton-Lycra knit
Cotton Gabardine	Cotton knit
Cotton twill	French terry
Lightweight denim	Georgette
Lightweight bull denim	Jersey knit
Lightweight poly-wool	Lightweight cotton
Linen	Lightweight gauze
Nylon techno-fabric	Matte jersey
Poplin	Novelty knits
Shantung	Nylon and nylon blends
Sheeting	Peachskin (a microfiber)
Tropical suiting	Piqué
Woven cotton/Lycra	Ponte knit/rayon blend
	Ramie/cotton
	Rayon
	Silk
	Terry cloth (active wear)

Winter	
Structured	**Fluid**
Corduroy	Acrylic and acrylic blends
Denim	Angora
Faux-fur	Cashmere
Flannel	Charmeuse
Gabardine	Chenille
Leather	Cotton-wool blends
Oxford cloth	Faux-fur—thick pile
Poly-wool	Fleece
Satin	Peachskin (a microfiber)
Velveteen	Pinwale corduroy
Vinyl	Poly-wool
Wool	Ramie/cotton
	Silk
	Suede
	Velour
	Velvet
	Wool

summer clothes. Remember, use the above list as a guideline. There are no set rules for fashion. I'm seeing light-weight, pastel-colored cashmere tops with cotton/Lycra twill capris for Spring/Summer. Soft, fluid fabrics like wool, can be lined and made into structured garments, so don't let this section scare you. There is no need to pack up your piqué shirt as soon as it gets crisp outside. Wear it under a leather jacket or light wool blazer for a smart, casual look.

Taking Care of Your Clothes with Mindfulness

Not long ago, my husband and I were reading a book on Buddhism. All throughout, the writer stressed one word over and over: "mindfulness." No matter what activity or task you are doing whether it is something artistic like designing or painting, or something as mundane as doing the dishes, when you do it with mindfulness it becomes an event that engages your whole self. I try to think about this when I'm designing my line but also when I'm caring for my clothes. Laundry is a chore, but I have to do it—it's a fact of life. So rather than going about it resentfully, I might as well try to enjoy it. I try to think, "If I treat my clothes with respect, if I am *mindful* of the way I care for them, they will last far, far longer. I can enjoy these clothes for years, and I won't rack up heavy dry-cleaning bills." So I don't just dump everything into the washer, run off, and return five hours later to bundle everything into the dryer on the highest setting. When it's time to do laundry, I try to take the time to be mindful of what I'm doing.

I'm a firm believer in using the delicate setting for almost everything you wash. If you have taken the time to shop carefully for your clothing and have chosen to spend your money on it, it deserves a little extra special treatment, don't you think? Wash your clothes on delicate with a little Woolite or mild soap. Don't run off and do a hundred other things while your favorite clothes are in the washer, it's too easy to forget them. When wet clothes are left sitting their colors can run, and the fibers can break down. If you leave them too long, your clothes can start to mildew. This is not mindful treatment.

I made a little lace lingerie-bag with a drawstring for my hose and underwear, which keeps the washing machine from eating them. I'll put them in on the delicate cycle with my other good clothes. When it comes time to turn them over to the dryer—set on "cool"—I keep my hose in the lingerie-bag so they won't get knotted and snagged. Lingerie bags are quite inexpensive and they'll add many more wearings to the life of your hosiery.

When you're doing your clothes, part of being mindful means finding a chore that will keep you at home near the washer and dryer. It's far better to take the clothes out of the dryer as soon as they are done. Not only is there something really satisfying about taking out a load of warm, clean, fresh clothes, but getting to your dried clothes quickly will prevent wrinkles and unnecessary ironing.

Certain garments should never go in the dryer. Wool and cotton sweaters should be blotted (never wrung, it will stretch the knit) and laid flat on a towel to dry. If you mistakenly put a wool or cotton sweater in the dryer, don't despair. Sometimes it can be salvaged. Rewet the sweater and stretch it out on a towel. Pin it in place, put another towel on top, and then something heavy to hold it down. It may come back. The same goes for other delicates. A woman I know thought she could get away without dry-cleaning her favorite black georgette skirt. It shrunk two sizes and she was devastated. She tried stretching the skirt on an ironing board and running a steam iron over it, letting the steam act as a dampener. It wasn't perfect in the end, but she stretched it back to a wearable state.

Dressing For the

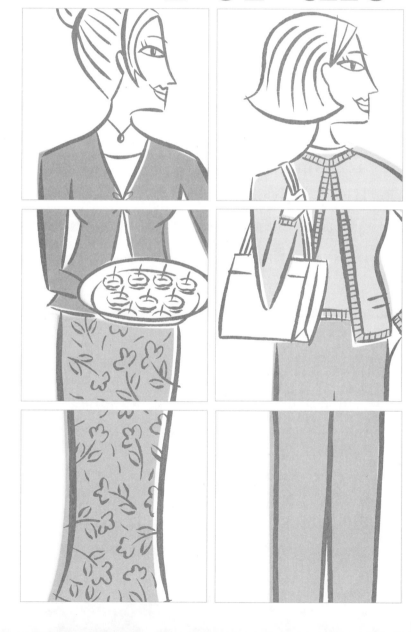

Chapter 6

Occasion

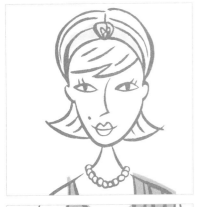

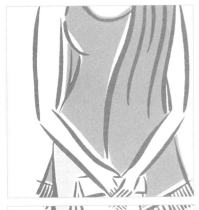

Dressing for an occasion is like dressing for a role. Your voice and what you say will ultimately tell people who you are and what you know, but it is essential to make a good first impression, whatever the situation.

If you've established a confident closet, you'll always have the pieces to put together a proper outfit for any occasion. The one exception might be a formal black-tie affair. Then it's time to buy something very special or make use of a simple black dress that can be elegantly accessorized.

Whatever the occasion, if you have to err on the side of being either underdressed or overdressed, I'd say go over-dressed. I think it's better to be the best-dressed woman in the room than to risk feeling inferior. I'm not saying that you should wear your evening gown to the PTA meeting, but only that you should take your time in choosing clothes to match your appointment or invitation. So here are a few ideas to get you thinking. You need to

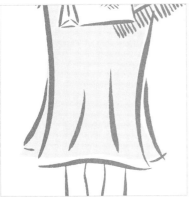

get in touch with your feelings and think about the way you want to look. What makes you feel pretty or makes you feel special? Would you prefer to cover your arms, or are bare arms flattering for you and appropriate for the occasion? Do you feel like wearing a dress or a pantsuit or perhaps a skirt and jacket? Do you look best in prints or solids? What colors make you feel most happy and alive? These are a few of the questions you must ask yourself before you begin to put together the perfect outfit.

What to Wear…

To a Corporate Office

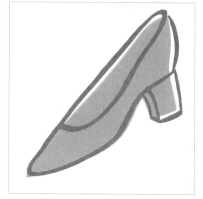

The corporate environment has truly evolved when it comes to women's style. A smart-looking, well-made skirt suit can make a very strong, serious impression. And a smart-looking, well-made pant suit can be just as powerful, even though I think that strong, confident, business women should not have to trade power for femininity. So just what is a serious suit? I believe it's dark, structured, and well-fitted, with a solid blouse or shell underneath. The jacket and trousers must have a basic traditional cut, nothing trendy. The skirt should either hit the knee or just below the knee, or be a mid-calf length, whatever looks best on you. A slim skirt looks more powerful then an A-line or dirndl. If you are in a conservative setting, opt for a wool gabardine jacket, fully lined, in a classic color. It doesn't have to be black, but it shouldn't be baby blue, either. Underneath the jacket, wear a tailored white shirt or an ivory shell—something neutral. I wouldn't go for a red shirt or a bright pattern. If you work in a corporate office, but have identified yourself as Fluid, why not look for a suit in a matte jersey knit? Peachskin suits can also fit the bill. As for shoes, look for a medium heel in a dark color. Carry a simple, well-made, and well-cared-for black leather clutch or bag with short shoulder strap. Opt for nude or dark hose that match both your skirt and shoes.

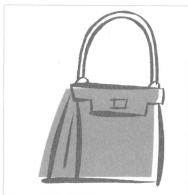

To a Job in the Fashion Industry or Advertising

Outside of the corporate environment, you have a lot more leeway with what you can wear to work. In certain professions, you are even expected to dress with an eye to the latest fashions—if for no other reason than to show you know what's in style. In these offices, you can get away with far brighter colors, garments with fashion flair, and less-than-classic trousers. You might carry an oversized purse or bag and wear platform shoes or mules if they work with an outfit. But the one thing I would not do is go kooky on makeup and hair. Even if bright orange lipstick and iridescent eyeshadow is the hot look, you still want to project professionalism. You want to say, "I know what's happening in fashion but I'm still in control." You want to be taken seriously, and you don't want someone to be distracted by your wild hair or makeup. I also wouldn't put on a trendy outfit that doesn't look good on you. If chartreuse is the biggest color, but doesn't suit your complexion, don't wear it. I had a meeting with a woman the other day who was wearing the most gorgeous outfit—she had on a sheer plum-colored peasant top with glitter studs over a tank top, and a silk shantung slim skirt. The clothes were stunning, but she was out of shape and the outfit looked too skimpy and trendy on her. It actually detracted from an otherwise beautiful sixty-five-year-old woman. The sleeveless blouse revealed tone-less, dimpled arms and the blouse did nothing to flatter her figure. She was trying too hard to look young, and strangely enough, the outfit aged her more. I'm all for style and trend, but it's got to be worn tastefully.

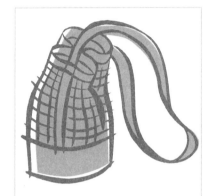

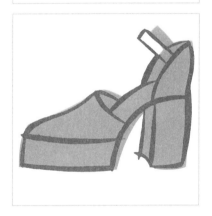

I also remember working with a designer who favored heavy, purple eye shadow and bright-colored wild prints in fluid fabrics. It was hard to take her seriously when all I could think of as I looked at her was her clown-like appearance.

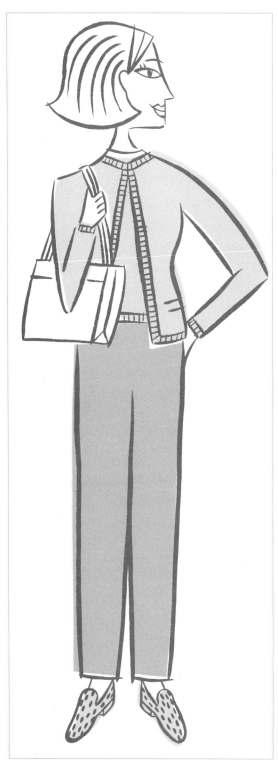

On Casual Friday

More and more offices have instituted casual Friday, a day at the end of the week where men can lose their ties and women can leave their blazers at home. But just because the day is called "casual," don't take it to mean "sloppy." You never want to show up for work looking like you've been running Saturday-morning errands and you just happened to stop into the office. Remember, you are still going to a place of business where you must dress appropriately. Aim to look casual but neat. I would suggest a sweater set with a pair of Lycra twill trousers. Forgo the jeans unless they are neat and fresh—nothing old and worn out. Colored jeans, such as black, olive, or khaki, always look smart, and the newest high fashions can be chic as long as they're not overdone. You can afford to wear fun and more comfortable shoes, but avoid tennis shoes, open-toed sandals, and flip-flops. Try a nice loafer, clog, or fashionable mule.

From the Office to the Evening

Here's where your black sheath comes in handy: take off the corporate jacket you wore over it during the day and add chunky pearls and a pair of high-heels you've brought in your black leather bag. Or start the day in a black tank top and a black slim skirt. In the evening trade your jacket for a lacy sweater and put on a fun necklace, strappy, sexy shoes, and carry a beaded handbag.

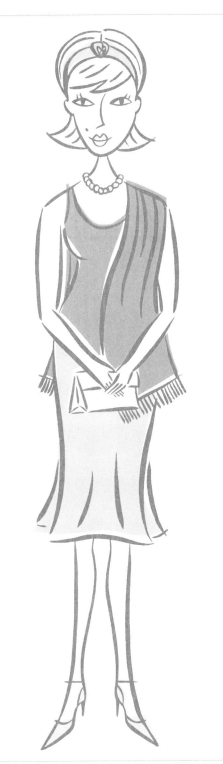

Leaving your tailored jacket behind, changing your shoes, and adding the right accessories will take you easily between office and evening when you don't have time to go home and change.

On a First Date

When you're going out with someone for the first time, you want to look confident without being intimidating. Don't overdo it. Keep your clothes, hair, and makeup simple but elegant. You want to let him know you are thinking about him—but maybe not too much.

Even if you're going to the movies, save the jeans for later. Choose nice tailored trousers with a casual shirt. Bring a light sweater in case the theater is chilly. If you prefer skirts, wear one that's not too short with a nice sweater or sweater set. If you're going out for dinner and dancing, wear a fun top, a flippy skirt that will move when you dance, nude or colored hose, and a higher heel. You want to look a little flirty but not too dressy. Don't wear jewelry that could fly off while you're dancing. Take a pretty wrap along instead of a coat.

To a Garden Party

A garden party calls for a light summer dress in a pastel or midtone. You want to pick up the color of the garden—the soft greens and pinks, the delicate blues. Unless you are in Hawaii with its vibrant tropical flowers, don't wear electric brights. Opt instead for something soft, flowing, and romantic. I would choose a fluid dress in a

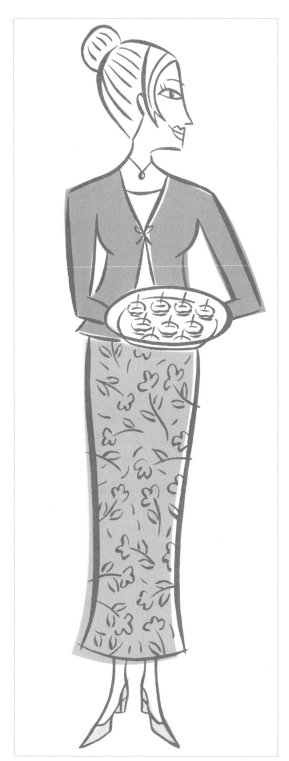

midcalf length—no boardroom power skirts here. If the party is going into the evening and you'll want to cover up, pair your dress with a light cardigan or shawl. If you prefer the structured look, choose a light linen dress or linen trousers with a nice cotton T-shirt. Keep the heels of your shoes low and wide. Spike or high heels will dig into the ground and pull off when you walk. Now's the time to wear your wide-brimmed straw hat to keep the sun off your face.

Entertaining at Home

You've spent a lot of energy making your home a lovely and welcoming place; your clothes should reflect that same care. I believe in lightweight, washable fabrics for entertaining at home—lightweight so that you don't get too warm if you are cooking, and washable for those inevitable spills in the kitchen. I would opt for a fluid fabric, like peachskin or matte jersey. It doesn't matter if you choose trousers or a skirt, but make sure the heel on your shoe isn't too high. You don't want to trip with a tray of drinks or the turkey platter!

Apple Picking in the Country

An autumn weekend getaway calls for comfortable broken-in jeans or corduroys, a cotton or cotton-silk turtleneck, a thick wool sweater, and a casual jacket. Here you can wear either sturdy boots or tennis shoes. Don't forget your hat and gloves. You can always take them off if you get too hot, but they are handy when the wind blows. And slather on the sunblock. Summer isn't the only time you can get sunburned.

To Meet Your Child's Teacher

When meeting the person in charge of a considerable portion of your child's day, you should appear serious but approachable. You want your child's teacher to feel free to talk to you honestly without feeling intimidated. If possible, I would leave the power suit at home and choose twill trousers with a conservative sweater or sweater set. Now is not the time to wear anything kooky or far-out. You want to look responsible and parental.

To the Office Holiday Party

Just as casual Friday is still a day at work, the office party is still a business function. You are going to have to work with these people after tonight, so don't choose anything too outrageous or sexy. It's fine to show a little more skin, but be discreet. Your black sheath, dressed up with nice costume jewelry, would be perfect here. Now is also the time for richer fabrics and colors like burgundy or forest green velvet. If you usually wear your hair down, scoop it up with a glittery barrette or dressy head-band. The key is festivity in moderation.

For a Day at the Museum

Start from the feet up. You are going to be on your feet all day and you must wear comfortable shoes—though I still would avoid sneakers, you might decide to go out for a nice lunch afterward. Once you've chosen the shoes, pair them with cotton or linen trousers and a button-front shirt. A light wool blazer would be a nice addition, but nothing too warm. You don't want to get hot in the museum and be stuck carrying your jacket around.

To an Afternoon Wedding

An afternoon wedding calls for a dressier suit or dress in a lightweight fabric like cotton, rayon, peachskin, linen, or silk, in a pretty color. Choose a blue, lavender, or pink. Steer away from black for the afternoon, as well as heavy fabrics like satins and brocades. Many brides are upset if their guests wear white. If you are in any doubt, avoid it. Heels should be medium to high. If the wedding is outside, follow the rules for a garden party and avoid stilettos or anything spiky. Chunky earrings and jewelry are great and small elegant handbags finish off your outfit. I especially like coordinating shoes with my handbag. This gives a complete, thought-out, fashionable look.

To an Evening Wedding

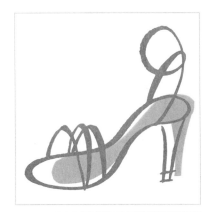

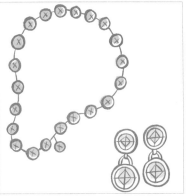

An evening wedding is the closest we come to a ball these days. If it's a black-tie affair, treat it as you would a gala and dress your most opulently. Choose a floor-length gown and go for glamour all the way. Rich silks and satins are appropriate , as are sequins and beading, but avoid heavy knits, wools, and sporty fabrics. Dress as glamorous as you like, but don't overindulge— too much glitz is overkill, and it can even be tacky and offensive. You don't want everyone staring at you when they should be looking at the bride. If you are wearing sequins or heavy beading, make sure that you don't overaccessorize. A sequined dress shouldn't have to compete with a rhinestone necklace. A small, fabulous purse is in order, big enough to carry only the essential—money and lipstick—and a pashmina or stole to drape over your shoulders if it's cold. I am a firm believer in simple elegance. There is nothing more striking than a long, simple gown with fabulous, strong accessories, or a gown in a flowing print or beautiful color worn with simple accessories. And last but not least, remember to wear elegant, dressy shoes that you can still walk and dance in. If you plan on dancing a lot, don't wear superhigh heels. Choose something gorgeous but comfortable.

To a Bar Mitzvah, Bat Mitzvah, or Christening

At any event that takes place in a house of worship, be respectful of your surroundings and don't show a lot of skin. For afternoon ceremonies, I prefer a simple tailored dress or a nice suit. A conservative skirt and a fitted or peplum jacket is a good choice. And I'd go for a lighter, more feminine color than a classic business suit. Soft ivory, pale pink, powder blue, navy blue, or silver gray can be stunning, especially if the fabric is a gorgeous silk, satin, linen, or shantung.

Of course, Bar Mitzvahs and Bat Mitzvahs are sometimes elaborate evening affairs. If they are black-tie, dress as you would for an evening wedding.

To a Funeral

I don't think you absolutely have to wear black to a funeral, though you do want to choose a dark, subdued color. Dark navy, deep brown, and charcoal grays are also appropriate. Make sure your clothing is conservative. Complete the outfit with dark hose, sensible shoes, and a cloth coat if you'll be outside at the burial.

When You're Pregnant

While not an occasion, pregnancy is certainly an event! It's possible to get through nine months of an expanding waistline on what you have in your closet if you play it smart. You might need to raid the father-to-be's closet once in a while or pick up a maternity dress if you are planning a special evening out, but on the whole you can get by with what you already own in the first half of your pregnancy.

When you first learn you are pregnant, look through your wardrobe and pull out anything in a dark color and anything with an elastic waist. Dark colors are slenderizing, and elastic waists will grow with you. Pull out any tunic top you have, any big shirt or oversize T-shirt. You should be able to wear your A-line dress up until the last couple of months. Many stores carry wonderful "pregnancy survival kits," containing a few coordinating pieces that are easy and comfortable to wear. You can also find upscale stores that sell adorable and fashionable maternity clothes that you can wear for a few months after the baby is born—since your figure may not come back for a little while. I for one didn't bounce right back to my prepregnancy weight. As a matter of fact, I still looked pregnant after my babies were born! Many women enjoy wearing Lycra leggings with big shirts or tunic tops even as new moms, and leggings provide both comfort and support.

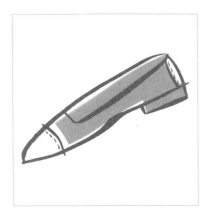

Do yourself a favor and don't buy any expensive item of clothing while you're pregnant—unless you have a special event where you must look dynamite—or anything in a fabric that can be ruined by the baby if you intend to wear it after you give birth. If you are going to breast-feed, stock up on button-front shirts. If you need a new bra, don't buy a regular one in a larger size, go ahead and buy a nursing bra even if you won't be nursing for a few more months. As a rule of thumb, if you buy clothes in the last two months of your pregnancy, think of choosing things you can wear for a year after your child's birth. It may take a little time for the weight to fall away and your waistline to come back.

The last thing to consider is shoes. Obviously, you want lower, sturdy heels and shoes with good traction, especially if you are pregnant during the winter and have to negotiate ice. Many women suffer from swollen ankles during pregnancy, so think about low boots to provide support and shoes with room to expand. Comfortable and colorful espadrilles are a good choice in the summer. Ballet slippers and Chinese shoes are great for around the house.

Use other mothers as a resource for swapping or borrowing clothes, so you won't be spending a lot of money on clothes that will swamp you in a year's time. Your new baby and all the accompanying paraphernalia will cost you plenty soon enough—so give your budget a break, while you can.

Shopping

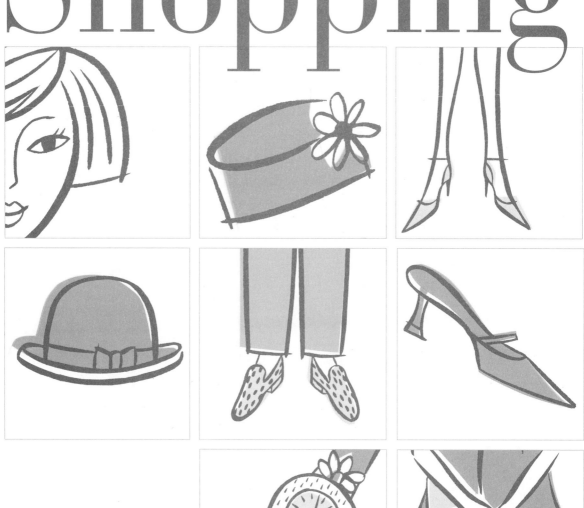

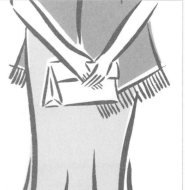

Chapter 7

I shop for a living. Two to three days a week, I am roaming department stores or scouring boutiques, scouting fashion trends.

I am forever flipping through catalogs and magazines. My life is so filled with shopping, you'd think I'd get sick of it. But the truth is I never do. I find shopping for the newest fashions exciting and invigorating. But I am so busy shopping and studying new designs for my work that I hardly have time to shop for myself. And I know that picking out clothes and finding the perfect fit can be a time-consuming chore. So here are a few tricks I've learned over the years, about where to go, and just as importantly *when* to go, to make sure you're getting the most for your money and time.

Where to Buy?...

While I'd love to believe you, and the whole world, buy only my clothes from my QVC show, I know your closet (like mine) is filled with items from all over. I can think of several main sources where women get their clothes: department stores, factory or designer outlets, specialty stores, discount stores such as Target and K-Mart, off-price stores such as T.J. Maxx, television, the Internet, and catalogs.

Each of these options has its good and bad points, and every woman has her favorite. I think the smartest shoppers draw from all these sources—and have the best wardrobes to show for it.

Department Stores

First, my little secret: I buy almost everything at an adorable specialty store in my neighborhood or at one of my favorite department stores. Even though I'm a fashion insider and know

how to get many things wholesale or make myself something, I rarely have the time to track down items and wait for them. It's easier for me to drive to the mall near my house which has one of my favorite stores—Neiman Marcus. Neiman Marcus carries top designers and the most up-to-date fashions and accessories. As a fashion designer, I prefer the newest items that hit the floor, and since I'm always in the stores shopping for new ideas, it's easy for me to spot what's new and exciting.

While I am inspired by fashion-forward looks when I design, I'm not one of those women who must have the most up-to-the-second-in-Milan style hanging in her closet. Although I love to be in fashion, sometimes I wait until later in the season to buy something when it goes on sale and it's a whole lot cheaper. Unless, I love something so much that I have to have it immediately, because it may be gone later, I try to wait. I never buy something unless I *absolutely* love it—I have too much experience buying "ho-hum" items that end up sitting in my closet. I only buy things that fit great and make me feel beautiful. Here are my reasons to buy things at full-price: you absolutely love something, it fits perfectly, and you can't live without it; you have an event the next day and no time to shop around; or you have enough money not to worry about price.

After years in the business, I have learned that department stores usually have two sales on any given garment, one half-way through its season—usually twenty percent off the tag price—and then another at the end of the season when they are clearing space for the next season's shipment—usually marked down another twenty percent. High-end department stores and specialty designer boutiques are usually a season ahead, which means they are selling designer spring fashions in February/March and designer fall fashions in July/August. They want to be out of their winter stock by November, because they need to move into cruise wear and the spring lines. If you can wait until the end of the selling season, which is the beginning of the real season, you can really save—often as much as forty percent off a garment's original price tag, which is almost its wholesale price.

Outlet Malls

By biding my time, I usually get as big a savings at a department-store sale as I would at an outlet store, but some people love the fun of devoting an entire day to outlet shopping and finding fabulous items at a fraction of the retail price. There is a wonderful strip of outlet stores near my vacation home in Vermont which features Tommy Hilfiger, Donna Karan, Calvin Klein, Ralph Lauren, Joan and David, Coach, Burberry, and Dana Buchman among others. But I know plenty of women who will drive hundreds of miles to a factory outlet when they could get the same deal at their neighborhood mall, but it's a treat to get out of town and hunt for bargains. It's often best to go outlet shopping when you have to buy a lot at one time—when your kids start school or you've switched jobs and need a new work wardrobe. You can often blitz the outlet malls and come away with deals that might have taken months to accumulate if you'd waited for department-store sales.

The garments you'll find at an outlet or factory store are usually returns, overruns, the result of a cancelled department-store order, odd sizes, leftovers from the previous season, and irregulars. It is far more important to check each item carefully for little flaws at an outlet than at a department store. A tiny rip in a seam you can sew up, a rip in the fabric means the item is garbage. Often, the outlet will point out a defect with a peel-off arrow or dot, but don't assume that's the only flaw. Check the garment thoroughly. If you are shopping in a department store's outlet, make sure the clothes aren't soiled or lipstick stained. Department stores ship end-of-the-season garments that haven't been snatched up in their sales to outlets, so they've been pretty pawed over by the time they get there.

I think the best things to buy at outlet malls are classic staples for next season. If you go to an outlet looking for the season's cutting-edge designs, you're already too late. And by the time you can wear that tie-dyed minidress again, it may be out of

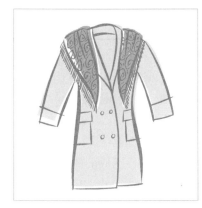

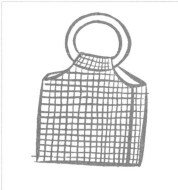

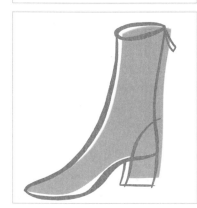

style. Instead, pick up a pair of denim shorts that you know you'll wear next summer, or a simple wool coat that you know will take you through next winter. Turtlenecks, classic blouses, suits, skirts, and trousers—things that hold up season after season—are good buys at outlet malls.

Discount Stores

It used to be that the only places to buy clothes were a department store or your local boutique. Then about twenty-five years ago places like K-Mart, Wal-Mart, and Target started popping up. These are called discount stores, and their prices are about twenty percent lower than a regular department store's. They buy in huge quantities and pay a lower wholesale price from the manufacturer and then pass the savings along to the customer. Sometimes they have their own labels such as K-Mart's Martha Stewart line, although designers must manufacture goods to meet the store's price point. Discount stores are great for buying children's clothes, lightweight garments like T-shirts and shorts, trendy items, or rugged items like blue jeans and denim jackets. You can buy accessories like handbags, hosiery, hair accessories, and fun costume jewelry.

Off-Price Stores

Say a department store has placed an order with a manufacturer and, for whatever reason, the store is having a bad season. Then the manufacturer calls and says they will be late delivering the shipment the store had ordered. If the store is in trouble, it will often use the manufacturer's delay as an excuse to cancel the order. Trust me, if the store needed the clothes, it would take them anyway, no matter how late. . . Now the manufacturer is stuck. They've produced all these clothes, but unless they own an outlet store, they have nowhere to sell them. That's when they call an off-price store. I have a real love-hate relationship with these stores. They have great savings because they have smart buyers who know the manufacturer is over a barrel. I've been the customer, but I've also been the manufacturer!

Off-price stores, more than discount stores, are where you can find some big designer names as well as lesser-known European designers. A woman I know found a famous designer's floor-length dress for ninety-five dollars that normally retailed for three hundred and fifty, and it fit her perfectly. She's already worn it five or six times; it's more than paid for itself.

Television

Television shopping is great for those of us with busy schedules. You can watch TV and shop while folding clothes or going over a business report and you don't have to pay for parking! You can pick out a new dress while preparing Thanksgiving dinner or buy a new business wardrobe from your StairMaster. Of course, because I'm a designer who sells through television, I may be biased. Still, I think it's an extremely convenient way to shop— especially when you can see live models moving in the clothes. We show the same item on models of different sizes and body types so that you can see how the clothes will look on you. We show different ways of wearing each item to suit different lifestyles. Pictures in catalogs are not only static, they also tend to be romanticized—young, beautiful girls walking on the beach or curled up by the fire, that sort of thing. It's sometimes hard to see how the clothes really look.

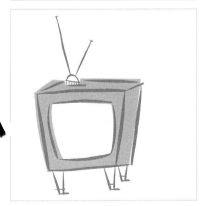

Many women use television shopping to create their own private dressing rooms. They can order a number of garments and try them on in the privacy of their homes. When you can't try on an item of clothing, it's extra important to know your measurements. After you identify a model with your body shape and see how the clothes fit her, use the size charts the show provides to determine what size to order. And when you call to place your order, feel free to ask the operator as many questions as you want about the garment and how it fits–that's what the operator is there for.

You need to be careful that you don't let a host's enthusiasm tempt you into an item of clothing that doesn't work with your overall wardrobe. I know I'm excited about every garment I produce, but if you bought everything I suggested, your closet would take over your house. Remember to shop as wisely through TV as you do elsewhere.

On shows like mine, you are often getting a price similar to what you would get at a discount store. Like a discount store, QVC buys in such large volume that they get lower wholesale prices. When you shop with me, what you get are up-to-date fashions—never last season's leftovers—including great basics and exclusive designs, and all without the hassle of fighting your way through the mall. It's truly a great convenience—QVC stands for Quality, Value, and Convenience!

I have become quite a QVC shopper myself. I buy jewelry, home items, beauty products, Legacy Legwear, hair products, toys, dolls—the list goes on! I am forever shopping the stores for new designs, so in my free time I try to keep out of the stores! It's a pleasure to purchase items that I need from the privacy of my own home and have them delivered. Now that's real convenience!

The Internet

The Internet is another great way to shop. Many Web sites, like our iQVC, have interactive screens where you can personalize your shopping by plugging in your measurements, your hair and eye color, your likes and dislikes—you basically build a computerized personal shopper! Once all your information is on file, some sites will even send you updates on new fashions that fit the profile of what you're looking for. At it's best, Internet shopping is convenient and fun. You can shop anytime, day or night, and have your clothes delivered, usually within days. At its worst, pictures take too long to download, and you have no more sense of the clothes than you would from a catalog. Take your time and surf. You'll soon find sites that work for you. And a little tip: most well-known stores and designers now have Web sites.

Catalogs

Catalog shopping used to fill a valuable niche before the advent of television and Internet shopping. They are convenient because they come straight to your house and are directly targeted to you based on your overall shopping patterns. Catalogs are lots of fun. You can flip through them in the bathtub in the evening or while your power shake is in the blender before your morning jog. I keep a stack of catalogs at my bedside and I go through them every night. I pull out pages of items I would like to order and then say to myself, "Just sleep on it." By the time morning comes I decide whether or not to go ahead and order the item. But catalogs are not as flexible as Internet sites, and they don't offer the motion and excitement of a television-shopping show. I'd say that if a company you already like sends you a catalog, buy from it. If a company is new to you, go on-line and see if they also have a Web site. Famous catalog producers like J. Crew and Victoria's Secret have sites. Use their phone operators if you are unclear about sizes and carefully check their return policies. But remember that you probably won't save money ordering by catalog—catalog prices are comparable to most department-store prices.

Thrift Stores and Tag Sales

I used to love going shopping for vintage clothing and accessories, but as my schedule got more hectic, I had to let it go. There are hundreds of hidden treasures in thrift stores and at tag sales across America, but you need a good eye and lots of time to sort through junk. If you have both, you can come away with gold.

What I would look for in a thrift store are things you can't find in a conventional shop—a unique print shirt, a beaded sweater, a fun piece of costume jewelry, or a really spectacular handbag.

If you take up vintage shopping as a hobby you can really spice up your wardrobe with original pieces and accessories.

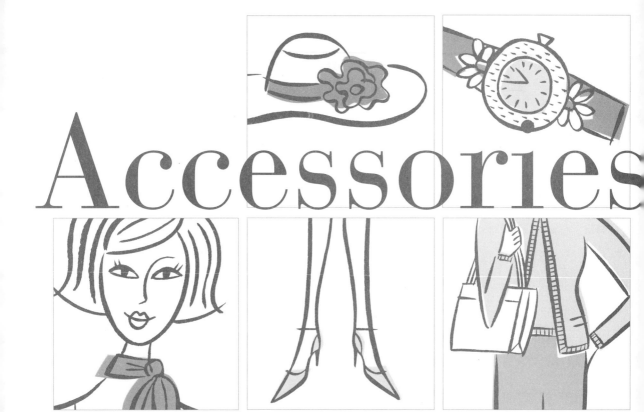

Accessories

Chapter 8

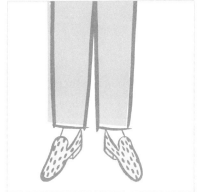

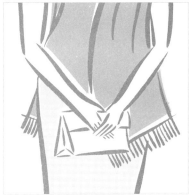

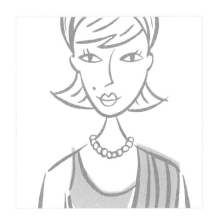

$\mathcal{A}$lthough I am a firm believer in accessorizing first with clothes, it's true that once your wardrobe is well rounded, it's great to have a wide range of accessories to complement your closet.

Traveling is a great way to pick up unusual accessories. Betty, who makes my patterns, brought me a little red silk bag from China. I treasure this beautiful bag and always get compliments when I carry it. When I was in London last year, I picked up a huge Scottish tartan that I can wrap around my whole body. It's incredibly warm, I wear it in place of a coat. It looks great with a skirt and boots or jeans and a heavy sweater. It's always smart to check out what women are wearing in Europe. If it's hot there, it's probably on its way here.

Wherever you go to find them, there are some accessories no confident dresser can afford to ignore. Let's start with the essentials—your shoes and handbag. Coordinating your shoes with your handbag will give you a super-polished look. So when you shop for shoes, ask yourself if you have a bag at home that will go with them—and vice versa, when you're choosing a bag.

Shoes

Shoes alone could fill a whole book, but we'll concentrate here on a few basic looks. I'm always amazed at how many career women, who are otherwise impeccably dressed, pay little or no attention to their shoes. If you walk through Grand Central Station in New York, you'll see dozens of men getting their shoes shined, but women are often walking around with scuffed leather and worn heels. Shoes complete your wardrobe, say a lot about your status in the world, and should be taken seriously. The wrong shoes can kill an outfit and perfect shoes can turn a good outfit into a dynamite outfit.

I don't think you need to spend a fortune on shoes, but make sure they fit. When your feet hurt you, your whole appearance suffers. Discomfort and strain from a pinching shoe show on your face and make you look tired and cranky. I often dress from my feet up. If I wake up tired, I won't put on those higher-heeled shoes. I'll wear something less challenging and opt for trousers that day rather than a skirt.

You can't do without a pair of classic black pumps. Choose a medium-high heel, and make sure they are in style—you don't want to wear a thin heel when chunky heels are the fashion. Buy them in leather to last longer, or cloth if the season allows. Besides your classic black pump, your complete shoe wardrobe should also include two pairs of casual shoes—such as loafers or oxfords, two pairs of dressy shoes—higher heels, slingbacks or straps, a pair of boots, and one or two pairs of sandals. Ten to twelve pairs will give you a complete shoe wardrobe. Instead of buying whatever crazy style is popular at the moment, why not experiment with color? You could rush out and buy a high platform wedge with a little mirror on the back, or you could buy a more classic style in red. Colored shoes are fun and different, and they won't go out of style. If you're going to wear high heels, you'll be more comfortable in a shoe with a slight platform in the front to lessen the angle of your foot. If you can only afford one pair of boots, buy them to fit a third of the way up the calf so that you can wear them under pants, and choose a medium-high stacked heel.

Make intelligent shoe decisions: work with the size and shape of your feet and the thickness of your ankles. I have thicker ankles, so I don't like to wear straps that call attention to them, and I like my shoes to be cut lower in front. If I do wear a strap, it crosses at the ankle to slenderize my foot. Wearing darker hose minimizes thicker ankles, just as darker shoes make big feet look smaller. If you have very large or wide feet, steer away from light-colored shoes because they will draw the eye down and accentuate the size of your feet. As a rule of thumb, I like at least a thin rubber layer on the soles for traction. I hate slipping in new shoes! It's a personal preference, but I also like the soles of my shoes to be dyed. If you are wearing a sandal, be mindful of your feet. Either get a pedicure, or simply keep your nails clean and neat. There is nothing less attractive than chipped nail polish with open-toed sandals. If you don't have time to repaint your toenails, take old polish off—or just stick to clear polish.

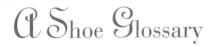

A Shoe Glossary

❋ Boot—extends anywhere from ankle to thigh

❋ Espadrilles: soft fabric shoe with flat woven sole

❋ Loafer: moccasin-like slip-on shoe

❋ Mary Jane: pump with strap across foot

❋ Mule: backless slip-on

❋ Oxford: low-heeled lace-up

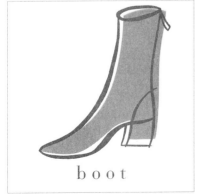

b o o t

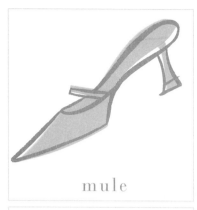

mule

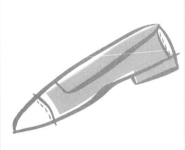

spectator shoe

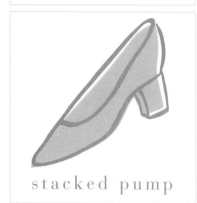

stacked pump

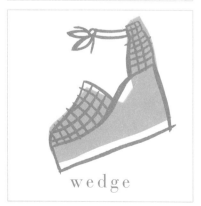

wedge

❋ Open-toed: cut out to expose the toe

❋ Platform: a thick sole under both toe and heel

❋ Slide: backless open-toed slip-on

❋ Slingback: strap around an open back

❋ Spectator shoe: two-toned, usually black and white, tan and white, or black and tan

❋ Stacked pump: thicker heel, usually built of layers of leather

❋ Stiletto: pointed, narrow high heel

❋ Thong: open flat shoe with straps across the toes starting from between the big and second toes

❋ Wedge: solid heel, heel higher than toe

Handbags

Nothing ruins a great outfit like a worn-out handbag. A mis-shapen, stained, or banged-up bag says that you don't really care about your total look, that you haven't taken the time to put yourself together. Luckily, there is no excuse for a bad bag. Discount and off-price stores sell great bags at great prices. With the bargains out there, you can have a bag for every mood and every season, as well as your practical everyday bag.

Your number-one purchase has to be a simple black bag. To my mind, the perfect bag is not too large and not too small—

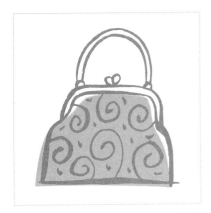

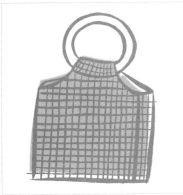

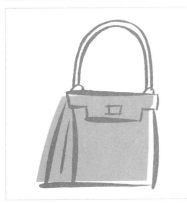

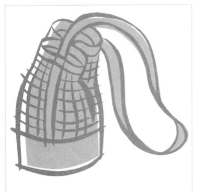

it's big enough to carry your wallet, checkbook, compact, lipstick, and cell phone. It should have straps so that you don't have to fumble with it when you're trying to get through a door or onto the bus. It can be leather or a washable fabric. A black bag is sophisticated and seasonless and goes with everything except the very dressiest outfit. Having a basic black bag will save you time, because you'll never have to worry about switching handbags to go with your outfit. Black works great with colors, solids, and prints.

I don't know what I'd do without my black bag. It goes everywhere with me and is essential to any wardrobe. The one I'm carrying now is a little on the expensive side—my daughter helped me pick it out, she's got great taste!—but I've had perfectly good black bags in the past that weren't expensive at all. I know that a lot of city women opt for smaller bags with straps that they can wear diagonally across their chests.

Handbag styles change from season to season, so besides the black bag, I like to have at least two or three seasonal bags. Again, it doesn't have to cost you a lot of money, and it's a great chance to add something cute and trendy for the season. For last spring and summer, I chose a hand-embroidered, natural hemp bag. It has a tortoise-shell handle and a drawstring to keep things from tumbling out. It's casual enough to wear with jeans and whimsical enough to pair with a dress. It's fun and flirty and very feminine. This fall and winter, I've been carrying a raspberry felt bag, decorated with beading and embroidery in a bouquet of different colors—yellow, light blue, brown, and pink. I can carry the handbag when any of these colors accents a color I'm wearing. Because it's small and classically shaped, it works well with almost anything from casual jeans to a traditional suit to an elegant silk dress. Whatever the outfit, the handbag is a stunning eye-catcher. I must admit to a passion for bags and shoes—they can make a tremendous difference to your outfit and appearance.

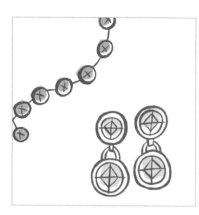

Jewelry

We all love jewelry, including me—even though, I believe jewelry is a secondary accessory. Only after you've put together accessorizing pieces of clothing—which will ultimately do more for your overall look—should you think about what jewelry to buy to best complement your wardrobe.

I am a big fan of jewelry that makes a statement, that's a little bit out of the ordinary. I buy jewelry a lot like I decorate—I look out for special, one-of-a-kind pieces that say something about me and what I like. If you favor the traditional look, go for classic pearl earrings, but you might want to choose something a little different, like a pearl with a drop. If you like unadorned metals, buy hoops in brushed pewter from a local artisan for a more distinctive look. If your tastes are more dramatic, look for interesting pieces from designers who combine gold and silver with beading. You could even rescue vintage pieces from your mom's or grandma's jewelry box. As the saying goes, "Everything old is new again!"

Earrings

The trend in jewelry today is bigger and bolder. I see yellow gold making a tremendous comeback with large, chunky beads, hoop earrings, and bangle bracelets all the rage. Gone is the minimalist look of the nineties to be replaced by the big, bold, beautiful look of today.

Earrings are usually the first grown-up piece of jewelry that little girls beg their mothers for. With me it was the exact opposite; my mother begged me to have my ears pierced. Or I should say bribed me. I remember I was in the third grade and my mother gave me fifty cents to have my ears pierced. She thought I should have them done before I got old enough to be afraid of the pain! She had waited so many years and lost so many clip-on earrings before she got the nerve to have her ears pierced that she didn't want the same thing to happen to me. (Today's kids are so brave, they're piercing everything!) As it turned out, I actually fainted when I got mine pierced. I was ashamed to cry because my friends were with me. Before I knew it, I blacked out for a few seconds, but at least it was over and done with. Fascination with earrings doesn't die with childhood; I know more than one woman who feels naked leaving the house without them. Because they frame the face, earrings can become an extension of your personality even more than a bracelet or necklace. When you're feeling sophisticated, you'll pull out your twenty-four-karat gold knots; when you're feeling young and carefree, you'll reach for colored Lucite flowers. With the way they can add sparkle and shine to your look and your face, it's good to have a broad collection of earrings to match both your outfits and your moods.

There are a few things to remember when you buy earrings:

❋ Many people have metal allergies, so if you have pierced ears and you can afford it, go with gold, gold-plated, or silver posts. If not, at least make sure the earrings are hypoallergenic.

❋ Choose earrings that complement your ears. If you have small earlobes, don't wear heavy pierced earrings that will stretch your holes. On the other hand, if your earlobes are large, tiny studs will look lost.

❋ Dangle earrings look best on women with long necks. Stud earrings are more flattering on women with shorter necks.

❋ A good set of medium-size pearl earrings are great for any occasion and will carry you from the office to an evening out.

❋ Match your earrings to your wardrobe. If you wear crisp, structured clothes, romantic filigree earrings won't work for you.

If you're the type who loves flowing velvet, keep away from abstract geometric styles.

✳ I like to see metals match, so gold earrings and a silver necklace look wrong to me.

✳ Store your earrings in a plastic box so that you can see what you have. It's too easy to forget about a pair that might be perfect with the outfit you're wearing.

✳ If you find you are always losing the backs to your earrings, check your local crafts store. They often sell boxes of extra earring backs.

✳ If you are out and you lose the back to a post earring try this trick: Break the eraser from the end of a pencil and use it to secure the earring—it really works well, I've tried it!

Necklaces

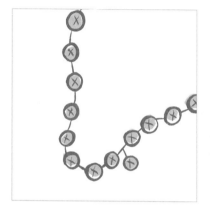

Next to earrings, necklaces are probably the most popular jewelry accessory. They can range anywhere from a simple serpentine gold chain to a multistrand beaded choker to a chunky strand of large crystals. I once bought my coworkers sleek, stunning, sterling-silver pens that hung from a cord, from Tiffany & Co. It was the perfect necklace for a woman who writes a lot on the job—beautiful, classy, and practical.

I think every woman should have one or two short necklaces, choker length to fourteen inches, and one dramatic pendant necklace that's at least sixteen to twenty-two inches long. A strand of pearls will take you through many of life's occasions. Pearls work at the office; they're perfect for a wedding; they even dress up the weekend's jeans and oxford-cloth shirt. Pearls don't have to be expensive. Many of the cultured strands available today are quite affordable. Black- and peach-colored pearls are very popular right now, and might fit the bill if you find classic white too sedate. I own a fabulous set of Judith Ripka faux pearls that I bought from QVC. They come in stations so that you can make them long or short or even double them. They also have a removable toggle that can transform the necklace to a bracelet. They are wonderful and truly elegant.

Here are some pointers to consider when shopping for a necklace:

✳ If you have a shorter neck, wear a longer necklace. You need a strand that falls just under the collarbone.

✳ A long necklace creates the illusion of height. A short necklace will make you look less thin and if you are very tall and thin, a choker will make you look shorter.

✳ If you have a long neck, layering different strands or wearing big, chunky necklaces can be quite elegant.

✳ Don't wear a short necklace with a turtleneck. It will get lost. Wear a necklace that falls below your collarbone, or even lower.

✳ If you have a full bust, make sure that you choose a long necklace with enough length to lie properly.

Why Not Experiment?

Necklaces aren't the only way to set off your neckline. Last season I bought a faux-fur collar, and I absolutely love it. It only cost me eighteen dollars, and it can really spice up an outfit. I wear it with anything, from a coat to a plain crewneck sweater. I snap it on, and voilà, my old black cardigan turns into high fashion. They make faux-fur cuffs, too, if you want a complete look. Next time you reach for another necklace or a scarf in the winter, try a faux collar instead—it's fun, chic, and fashionable.

Watches

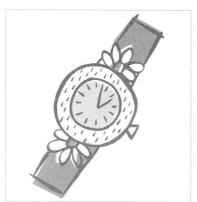

Everyone needs a watch. The kind of watch you choose says a lot about who you are and your lifestyle. Are you the sporty type who goes for a high-tech digital? Are you a classic Rolex wearer? Do you have a box of multicolored watchbands that you can coordinate with any outfit? A watch does more than tell time, it shows the world how you like to spend yours.

A few words about watches:

❋ If you wear a watch with a metallic band, choose one that goes with the majority of your jewelry. So if you wear mostly silver necklaces and earrings, don't buy a gold watch.

❋ If you wear a leather band, rub it with mink oil every now and again to prevent cracking.

❋ Experiment with older watches—but remember you need to wind them! One of my favorites is a watch I own that was my grandmother's from the 1920's. I treasure my "estate" watch, and I'm thankful that my mother gave it to me without even warning me not to lose it! It's a classic—and I've noticed that Cartier has come out with a similar style. Another watch that I wear was my husband's years ago. I've updated it with a bright-red leather band. It's fun to wear in the summer and its unusual, pulsating face is a real conversation piece.

I love watches and I never leave the house without a watch to match my style that day. From sporty to whimsical, traditional to dressy—I have one for every mood.

Hosiery

Once upon a time, all women wore individual stockings hooked to a garter belt. Then in the sixties, panty hose were invented and we were liberated! Now there is an infinite variety of hosiery, from silky sheer to textured colors to ribbed cotton. When the weather gets warm, I think it's fine to go stockingless. I used to think that hose were necessary to finish off an outfit, but I've changed my mind. More than ever, I'm seeing women looking absolutely stunning bare-legged in the summertime. And there are so many gorgeous open-toed shoes and sexy mules that call for bare legs. I think bare legs in the summer are totally acceptable as long as your toes are manicured and your legs look great. An adorable young friend of mine showed up at a summer afternoon Bar Mitzvah in a gorgeous dress and strappy sandals that worked perfectly with the dress. She is a beautiful girl with a figure to kill. Her mother thought her bare legs were totally inappropriate and was angry at her. I thought she looked much more chic than half the women there who were in pastel beaded suits or frilly dresses with dark hose and clunky shoes.

Here are a few rules of thumb for hose:

❋ I am a big fan of sheer darks and sheer nudes, and I'll choose them whenever possible. To me, white hose will forever be nurse-like and unflattering to a heavier leg.

❋ If you are showing a lot of skin on top—for example, you're wearing a strapless dress—wear nude hose. Dark hose will make you look bottom-heavy; nude will balance your look.

✳ Wear sheer black or nude hose when you're dressing up your black sheath.

✳ Avoid hose that are a lot darker than your skirt. Never wear black hose with a white skirt.

✳ Let the hose match the shoe. If you wear white shoes with dark hose, you'll look like Minnie Mouse. A monochromatic look is far more sophisticated and will make you look taller. Sheer chocolate brown hose with chocolate brown shoes is very elegant.

✳ Fishnet stockings and print or novelty hose can be fun for fall when worn with the correct outfit and shoes. But this look can be hard to pull off fashionably, so be very selective.

✳ Be careful choosing the fit. Too large and your hose will bag around the knee, too tight and you'll feel cut at the waist and crotch.

✳ Take great care washing and drying your hose; it will make them last longer. You can use a small delicate-laundry bag made of netting or lace, which lets you toss your hose in the machine so that you don't have to hand wash them. (If you're like me, you're always pressed for time.) This way they won't twist or snag. Set the machine on the delicate cycle. It's best to hang up your hose to dry, but if you don't, you can put them in a cool dryer as long as you keep them in the laundry bag to protect them from snagging.

Lingerie

Make sure your undergarments fit well. If you are small-chested, you may want a little padding to fill out an outfit, but don't overdo it. I prefer a natural look, no matter what your body type is. Small is beautiful, just as big is beautiful. As long as you are wearing clothes that suit your body type, your undergarments only need to fit well and be comfortable.

Make sure your bra isn't too tight; if it is you could end up with bulges at the shoulders or back. The same thing goes for your underpants; they should fit comfortably, and the elastic shouldn't be too binding. If you need support in the tummy, hip, or thigh try control-top panty hose, either over or instead of underpants. I also like the Legacy Body-Shaper Longline Brief from QVC. It's great if you need some support, but you don't want to wear hose.

Hats

With the recent studies on harmful UV rays, women have once more taken to wearing summer hats. Look for a hat with a brim that flatters your face. You may have to try on dozens, but I guarantee, you'll eventually find the perfect hat to light you up. Choose straw or canvas in the summer, faux fur or wool in the winter. If you are a woman who has battled cancer, you know how much better a pretty hat or turban can make you feel. Hats can be both the salvation of your skin and a fun way to complete your look.

I really love hats and own a small collection. A great hat can give a woman a very sophisticated, hip look. I always take notice of a woman wearing a fabulous hat and wish more women would wear them. How about we revive an old trend and all go out and buy sensational hats? I'll do it if you do!

Gloves

It used to be that a lady couldn't leave the house without her gloves. By the sixties and seventies, most women wouldn't be caught dead in them. Now, gloves have staged a comeback, and they're not just for winter anymore. Gloves are an elegant addition to almost any outfit.

Which Hat Is Right for You?

Come on! You don't look silly in a hat. Try different styles until you find the one that best flatters your face.

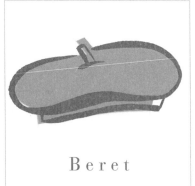

Beret

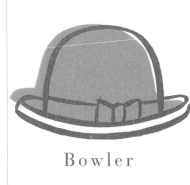

Bowler

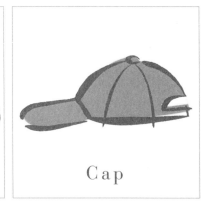

Cap

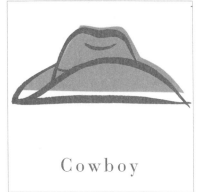

Cowboy

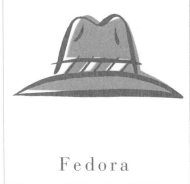

Fedora

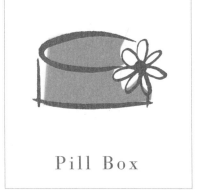

Pill Box

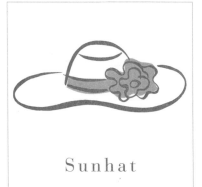

Sunhat

Like the basic black bag and pumps, a pair of black leather gloves is a must-have. Make sure the fingers are long enough to fit your hand and that they are not too tight around the palm. If winters are cold where you live, get them with a thin fleece or cashmere lining for extra warmth—but don't use your good gloves for scraping snow off the car. Keep a pair of thick wool mittens for that.

It's also good to have one or two pairs of "novelty" gloves. They could be stretchy leopardskin, chenille, or olive green leather—anything fun and fresh to brighten up the black coat you're sick of wearing by late winter. They're also great with a colorful wool sweater when it's just getting cold in the fall.

Scarves

Scarves are the perfect accessory for combining style and function. They can keep you warm in winter or accent your neckline like a necklace. I use scarves to add a touch of color to a classic, dark, business suit. There are millions of gorgeous scarves out there, in a variety of shapes, textures, and colors. Experiment with different styles and methods of tying, and see how dramatically a scarf can change your look.

How to tie a scarf

Square, sheer scarf:
Fold it in a triangle, fold the point down and roll it loosely. Tie it around your neck in a square knot and let the ends fall softly open. I like to wear the knot a little to one side. If it's in the front, you'll look too much like a Boy Scout!

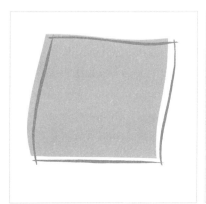
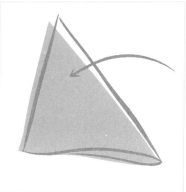

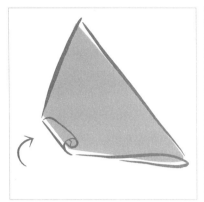

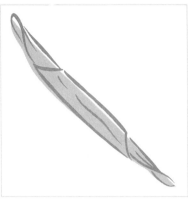

Big square, opaque scarf:
You can wear a big square
many ways. Tie it at the back,
cowboy style. Knot it off to
the side, or bring the ends
around and tie it in the front.
Drape it over your shoulders.
Wrap it around your neck like
a turtleneck.

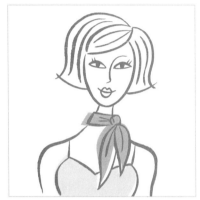

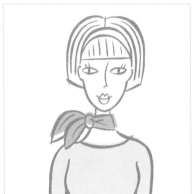

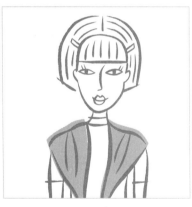

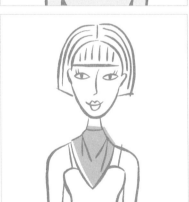

Long rectangular, sheer scarf:
Mine is transparent silk with
appliqué and beading. Pair it
with a strapless or spaghetti-
strap dress. Drape it across
your neck so that it hangs
down the back.

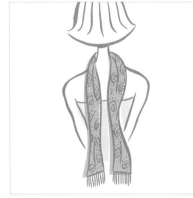

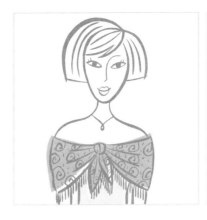 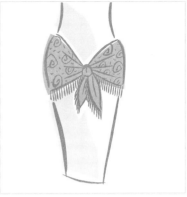

Triangular, silk scarf with beaded fringe: This is my favorite scarf. Mine is multicolored, in deep, rich colors with a heavy, beaded fringe—giving it a gypsy look. I tie it around my hips to dress up a long slim skirt. I wear it shawl-style with a dress. I wrap it around my shoulders and knot it in the front. The beading helps it stay in place and is also totally elegant.

❋ Be careful rolling a scarf. If you roll it or knot it too tightly, it will look like it's choking you. If you roll it too loosely, it could look too thick.

❋ Choose your scarf style carefully if you have a full bustline. For example, the cowboy look could emphasize your chest so much that it makes you look heavy.

❋ If you have a short neck or are Fan-shaped, avoid scarves. They will make your shoulders look broader and make you look stocky.

❋ If you are Bell-shaped, scarves are for you! They call attention to your upper body and away from your hips.

❋ Scarves look fabulous worn loose and flowing—not too carefully arranged and symmetrical. A great touch of color and class.

❋ Shawls and pashminas are wonderful additions to a wardrobe. I use them to add color and shine to an otherwise ordinary outfit. Recently my mother knitted me an open-mesh, long, gray shawl using hairy and metallic yarns intertwined. It looks rich and exciting across my shoulders when I'm wearing a basic dress and it adds sparkle to a classic suit. It's easy to find gorgeous embroidered scarves, with velvet, plaid, and pleated scarves for winter and magnificent florals year round.

The Total
Picture:

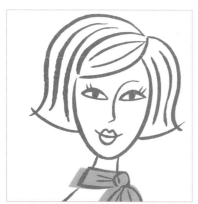
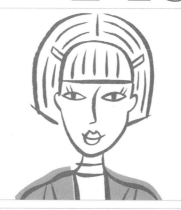
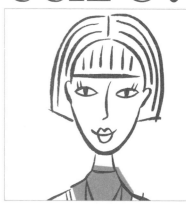
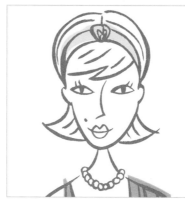
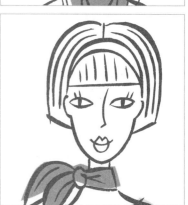
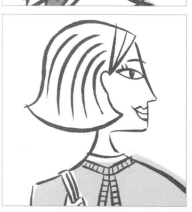

Chapter 9

Hair and Makeup

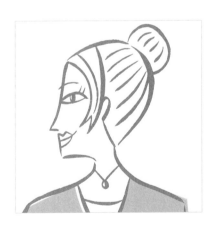

I don't claim to be either a hairstylist or makeup artist, so the advice I'm giving in this chapter is based solely on personal experience—but it's the experience of a woman who has been made up for television at least once a week for over ten years!

I can recommend some great books. Nick Chavez, a fellow QVC personality, has recently come out with a gorgeous and very thorough book on haircare and styling called *Perfect Hair Every Day*. There are also tons of beauty books available at your local bookstore, and you can always consult the person at your favorite department-store makeup counter or your regular hairstylist.

What I do know for certain is that hair and makeup play an essential part in your overall look. Nothing ruins a perfectly put-together outfit like shaggy or straggly hair. And you can be wearing the most expensive clothes in the world, but if your makeup is overdone and cheap looking, your overall look will be dragged down. It's pointless to spend a lot of money on your wardrobe only to ruin your look by neglecting your hair and makeup.

I personally think every woman looks better with a little concealer, blush, lipstick, and mascara. Even if you like the fresh-faced, natural look, a little makeup and light lipstick will make you look healthier. A rule of thumb: the more sophisticated the outfit, the more sophisticated the hair and makeup. You don't want to put on your expensive, tailored suit and then leave the house with a naked face and your hair pulled back in a pony-tail. On the other hand, heavy eye shadow, blush, and dark lipstick might look out of place with jeans and a casual sweater.

Your Makeup Bag

It's a good idea to invest in a nice makeup bag. Get one a little bigger than you think you'll need, to keep delicate shadows and powders from knocking together. When it's time to apply your makeup, take out only what you need and set it out in clear view. Arrange it in the order it goes on: concealer, foundation, powder, eyeliner, shadow, blush, lipstick. That way you can speedily work your way down the line. Be sure to apply makeup using a brightly-lit mirror or standing at a window with strong, natural light. This will ensure that you do not overdo it. Makeup should not be seen—it should enhance your beauty or cover any flaws. Putting on your makeup, except for the most elaborate occasions, should take ten to fifteen minutes at the most. It might take you longer if you're not used to wearing it, but with a little practice you'll get the hang of doing it quickly.

Whatever your outfit, the most important thing to remember about makeup is to keep it simple and appropriate. You don't want to look at a woman and see makeup, you just want to see a pretty face.

Skin

Good skin care is the first step in establishing a successful make-up routine. Every night before I go to bed I wash my face after taking off my makeup. My makeup artist at QVC has wonderful pads for removing eyeliner and mascara. They are not too oily and are very soothing. She also has a terrific foaming face wash that I use every night. It's a little minty and tingles on your skin. I swear by her products. After my skin is clean, I apply a separate eye moisturizer and face moisturizer. In the morning, I wash my face again and re-apply my eye and face moisturizers. I've been told that exfoliating is very important. I do it from time to time when I remember or have a free minute—which is hardly ever! But I think the most important thing is to keep your skin well moisturized and protected from the sun. When I was young, I used to bake at the beach, and now I'm seeing the damage.

I first begin with a good undereye concealer. Concealer covers a multitude of sins, from dark circles to small blemishes, and makes you look bright eyed and younger. Find a nice, creamy one, a shade or two lighter than your foundation. Make sure it's not too yellow, or it will make you look sallow. A concealer that doesn't complement your foundation will give your face too much contrast. And if you overdo the concealer, you'll end up looking like a raccoon. Be careful not to use a concealer that's too dry—many are—because if you're like most women, you have fine lines under your eyes. A concealer that's not creamy enough will make fine lines more noticeable. Use your concealer on your lids as well as under your eyes. If you don't have time for foundation and full makeup, make sure you remember to wear your concealer.

After the concealer, I apply a creamy foundation that matches my skin tone; I smooth it on with a triangular makeup sponge. I work with upward sweeps and make sure to blend it into my hairline and under my chin. Choose a foundation that's good for your skin type. If you have oily skin, find a product that keeps the sheen down; if your skin is dry and you are prone to wrinkles, find one with time-release moisturizers. Finish by lightly patting on a bit of translucent powder to set the foundation. Don't use too much or you'll end up looking cakey.

Eyes

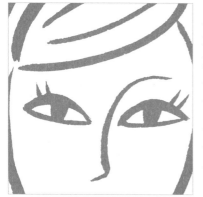

After my foundation is set, I move on to my eyes. Instead of a harsh pencil, I use powdered eyeliner applied with an angled brush. I like a dark chocolate brown because I've found black is too severe, especially for women with light eyes. Don't overdo it. You might think more eyeliner will draw attention to your eyes and make them look bigger. Actually, heavy eyeliner overpowers your eyes and makes them look smaller. Never take your eyeliner to the corners of your eyes, just use it in the middle.

Eye shadow comes next. Here too, I prefer a natural look and choose colors that work with my skin tone. I put a darker color, sometimes the shade of my eyeliner, in the crease of my lid to give the eye depth. Then I take a flat brush and apply a light beige shadow or the same translucent powder I used to set my foundation between the eyeliner and the eye shadow in the crease. This dot of lighter color in the center of the lid really opens up the eye. Finally, apply a little of the powder just under the eyebrow bone and right at the outside corner of the eye. All these touches will make your eyes look larger.

Mascara is the last thing I put on—and I like a lot. Sometimes I curl my lashes to make my eyes seem larger and more open. And don't neglect your eyebrows. You can buy an eyebrow gel that comes with a wand, like a mascara applicator, which will keep them tidy. Or in a pinch, you can use a bit of hair gel applied with a clean toothbrush.

Eyebrows

Don't go out with ragged-looking eyebrows. Bushy brows are as out as pencil thin, drawn-on brows. Today's look is a clean line that follows the curve of the bone structure beneath the eyebrow. The natural arch of your brows is revealed by plucking any stray hairs that might be lurking below the brow line or between your eyes. You can use your powdered eyeliner to gently feather in a little color to add definition. But remember, never pluck your eyebrows right before a big date or an important meeting because they can stay swollen and red for several hours afterwards. I like to have my eyebrows waxed; it's fast and they come out perfectly.

Cheeks

Blush is one way to simulate that healthy, outdoorsy look most of us women can't get from our busy, indoor lives. Make sure your blush is appropriate for your skin tone. If you want to give yourself cheekbones, take a little of your brown eye shadow and brush it under the apple of your cheek with a contour brush. Then smile when you apply your pink blush, brushing it just on the apple above the brown shadow. Blend, blend, blend. The brown simulates a true shadow, making your cheekbones look stronger. You can also strengthen your jaw or chin in the same way. Brush some brown eye shadow just below the jaw line or just under the chin to make either feature look more defined. You can also use brown shadow to make your nose appear smaller by applying it to each side of the nose.

Lips

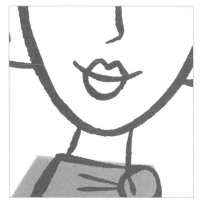

While I match my foundation and eye shadow to my skin tone, I coordinate my lipstick with my outfit. If I'm wearing something dark and muted, I'll go with a coral or a pink tone. If I'm wearing bright colors, I'll usually choose a more neutral lipstick that doesn't fight with the color of my outfit. Still, it's not a science. Sometimes a brightly colored outfit washes me out and I need bright lips to balance the look. But usually, I go for a more natural look and find I look best in softer corals and pinks.

Lip pencil is wonderful for defining the shape of your mouth. You can create the illusion of larger lips by applying the pencil just outside your natural lip line. If your lips are full, you can make them look smaller by drawing the line just inside your lip line. Choose a liner that matches the color of your lipstick. I use one just a shade darker than my lipstick and blend. Liner shouldn't be seen. It's like a girdle, it should be worn to give you shape and definition, but you should look as if you aren't wearing it.

In general, matte lipstick wears better than gloss, but I like the shine gloss gives you. Many makeup artists blot the lips with powder to set the lipstick so that it stays on longer.

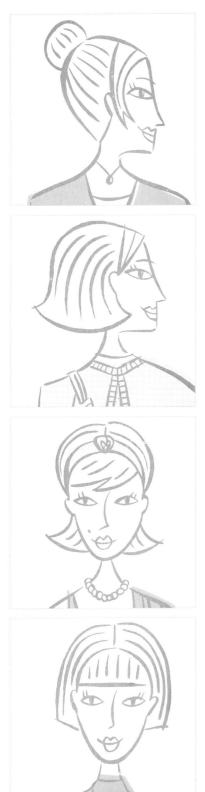

Hair

I love the look of long, flowing hair, but I always take notice of a striking short hairdo. Whatever your style or cut, healthy, well-groomed, natural-looking hair is absolutely essential to the success of your overall look. No matter how great your clothes are, if your hair is a mess, if your roots are showing, or your bangs are too long, you won't look good. Dull, brittle, or overprocessed hair is a sign that it's starving for tender loving care. As with the care of your clothes, be mindful of the care of your hair. Get it cut every five to six weeks, seven if it's just a trim. Make sure it is well conditioned, I like to get a végétal regularly, which is a process that leaves the hair looking healthy and shining.

The best choice for most of us is a natural-looking cut that doesn't require hours of styling. I'd steer clear of any cut so elaborate that it will cost you a fortune in visits to the salon just to maintain it. On the other hand, I wouldn't recommend a dreary all-one-length style that will drag down your face and make you look outdated. There is no hard and fast rule about what sort of hairstyle looks best on what sort of woman. If you have a small face and want to wear long hair, give it a try. If your face is long but you don't want bangs, that's fine too. Just don't be haphazard about the style. Talk with a professional stylist and ask about how you can get the most from your choice.

On a bad-hair day try some gel and pretty hair ornaments such as a headband or clip. Sometimes a simple pony tail will work. Some women look stunning with their hair slicked straight back. Not everyone can pull it off, but if you can, it's the perfect answer to a bad-hair day. My mother-in-law, Audrey, often slicks her hair back on a bad-hair day or if she is just in a hurry. She adds a beautiful bow at the back of her neck and looks totally elegant.

Packing

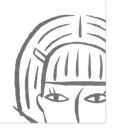
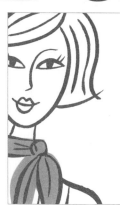
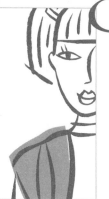

Chapter 10

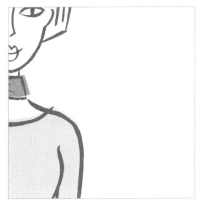

When I told my husband I was writing a chapter on packing efficiently, he looked puzzled and said, "I didn't think this was supposed to be a work of fiction, Susan."

Richie knows me too well! I'm a notorious overpacker, always throwing in that extra pair of shoes just in case we go to a fancy restaurant, or that fleecy jacket in case the weather suddenly plummets thirty degrees. But for the purposes of this chapter I want you to do as I say, not do as I do. (I might even try to heed my own advice. "Sure. . ." says Richie.) There is an art to packing and if you master it, you'll never worry again about giving yourself a hernia trying to shove your hundred-pound overnight bag into the overhead compartment. You'll have all the clothes you need and plenty of room to take home those little extras you pick up on the road.

Tips for Flying

I like to be comfortable on a flight, but it's important to be stylish even when you're traveling. I would chose a loose-fitting trouser in a soft microfiber or jersey knit—no tight jeans or short skirts. I don't know about you, but I always feel vaguely vulnerable when I'm going someplace new, and I want to feel confident and on top of my game when I get there. I pay a little extra attention to my hair and makeup, choosing simple, natural colors that I can touch up before we land. I wear my hair down or in a loose ponytail so that a barrette doesn't poke me when I lean my head back. I like to wear a lightweight cardigan, even in warmer months, because you never know if it's going to be cold on the plane. In my carry-on bag, I make sure I have fashion magazines to read, breath mints, a little bottle of lotion, and a small makeup bag. (You know that you should always pack all your medications, your glasses, and anything else you couldn't be a day without, in your carry-on.)

Core Groups

The first thing you must do before you start packing is identify the purpose of the trip. Now this seems really obvious, but take a minute to do it. There are many variables that go into dressing while you're away, and to pack efficiently, you need to determine which ones will dominate any given trip. Is it going to be solely a

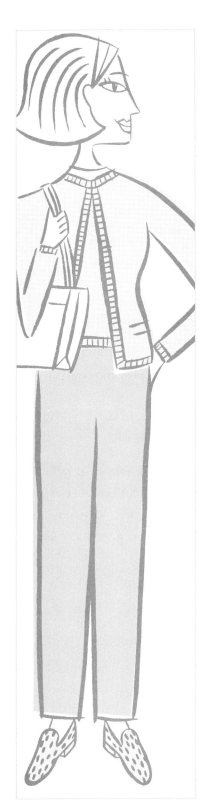

business trip with no other events besides meetings? Will there be dinners you'll need to attend? Will you have a day to yourself to do a little sightseeing? Is this a vacation, and if so, have you checked the seasonal weather charts for where you're going? Is it a combination of a business trip and a vacation, and if so, how many days will you spend on each? Whether the trip is primarily for business or pleasure will determine your core group of clothes.

If you have built your wardrobe wisely, you won't have any problem putting together two separate, but coordinating, core groups: one for business and one for pleasure. Each core group consists of five pieces around which you can add items and accessories depending on your activities. Make a list of your core pieces so that the next time you go away, you won't have to plan your packing all over again!

What Goes In

For each core group, pick a color scheme and stick with it. For business, black is often best. It's smart and sophisticated and doesn't show dirt, which is important if you need to wear the same pieces more than once. Black is also versatile; it can be jazzed up with a red scarf or a light blue shell. If navy or gray is your base color, go with it. Your business core group will reflect your Five Easy Pieces. Your vacation core group is more flexible. Still, the goal is to get the maximum number of outfits from the fewest items of clothing.

To these core groups, you can add pieces as the trip requires. You will obviously need several tops, but once you've established your dominant color, you can select tops that will go with everything in the group. You will need to choose appropriate shoes as well. A pair of classic black pumps will match everything in your Business Core Group. You'll probably want to include sandals and sneakers to go with your Vacation Core Group.

Business Core Group	Vacation Core Group
Dominant color: Black	Dominant color: Blue
One black slim skirt	One pair casual blue trousers
One black lined jacket	One blue skirt
One black pair of trousers	One pair blue shorts
One black sheath dress	One blue print sleeveless top
One white tailored blouse	Sundress
	One white T-shirt, long- or short-sleeved, depending on the weather

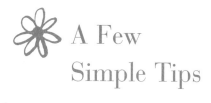

A Few Simple Tips

Here are a few examples of trips you might take and how you can pack using your two core groups.

Weekend At the Beach

Make sure the items in your Vacation Core Group are of cotton or some other soft fabric that will feel good against skin that might have gotten a little sunburned. You can use your sleeveless sundress as a beach cover-up, or you can bring a sarong or big blouse. Pack:

❋ Your Vacation Core Group

❋ Two bathing suits, so that one is always dry

❋ One light cotton sweater for evening

❋ One pair of nice sandals for going out, one pair of flip-flops for the beach

Three-Day Business Trip

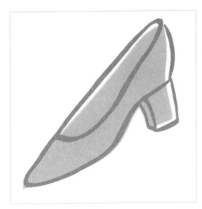

You will be in meetings most days, but you'll take the client out to dinner once and will have half a day to yourself for sightseeing. You should pack:

❋ Your Business Core Group

❋ One pair of stacked pumps, one pair of oxfords or loafers for sightseeing and your travel day

❋ Costume jewelry to take your black sheath from the board room to dinner

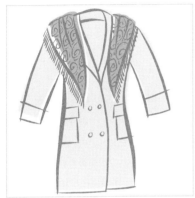

❋ Your black coat if it's cold

❋ If the hotel has a pool, you might want to pack a bathing suit and cover up.

Two-Week European Tour

First things first—take enough underwear! You don't want to get stuck doing a bunch of hand-washing or come back to your hotel to face a line full of dangling lingerie. This is supposed to be a vacation! If you are going to be away from home for a long time, you should double or triple your Vacation Core Group. Still stick to your dominant color, though if you'll be away for a long period, you might have to choose more than one dominant color. And remember—unlike underwear—you can wear clothes several times without washing them. If you are taking more than one of any given item, go for variety. For example, of three skirts, pack two long and one short.

For a long trip, I would pack lighter-weight fabrics, even in the winter, and layer. I'd rather take a thin cashmere sweater

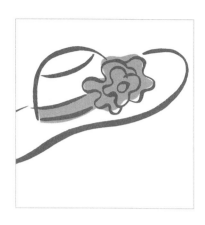

than a big chunky sweater. And obviously, adjust your core group to the weather. Keeping this in mind, pack:

❋ Your Vacation Core Group times three

❋ Three lightweight sweaters

❋ Your black sheath from your Business Core Group

❋ Three pairs of shoes: sneakers, sandals, and one pair of medium-heeled pumps for dining out.

How It Goes In

I've found a way of packing that keeps clothes virtually wrinkle free—let's face it, when you arrive at your destination after a long trip, the last thing you want to do is deal with pressing your clothes. There is always the old steam-them-in-the-bathroom trick, but that requires running the hot water for fifteen minutes or more and letting your garments hang in the steamy bathroom until the wrinkles drop out. It's wasteful, and it leaves your clothes limp.

Instead, I head off the problem by packing carefully. I know some people recommend rolling your clothes, and that works for microfiber skirts and thin T-shirts. Rolling sweaters and trousers, though, makes them bulkier, which means they take up precious room. Other than knits and microfibers, I don't fold or roll anything. Instead, I lay each piece of clothing flat, stacking as I go. The only garments I ever fold are trousers, because they are long. I first fold them at the creases and then in half, and place them at the bottom of the suitcase. Next I'll lay my sweaters and blouses flat, with the arms draping over the sides of the suitcase. You can even do this with suit jackets if you don't want to take a separate garment bag. Skirts are also laid out flat, or folded in half if they are long, and placed on top of the blouses. When you've got all your clothes in, carefully fold the arms of the blouses and sweaters and jackets over the stack—it looks like they have their arms folded over their chests. Lay your toiletry bag carefully on top along with your shoes, which should always be in cloth shoe bags or plastic bags, so they don't dirty your clothes. Try this method the next time you travel. Believe me, you'll never need a travel iron again.

When you reach the hotel, it's always a good idea to completely unpack and put your suitcase away. It will help with wrinkle control, and you won't be tripping over an open, disorganized suitcase. If you are lucky enough to be bringing only microfibers or knits, your packing will go much easier. These fabrics hardly wrinkle, and they are very lightweight—they're great for traveling. When you get to your destination, hang them up and any wrinkles should fall right out.

Accessories for Traveling

As with everything else, less is more when traveling. You want to take a few versatile accessories that can dress up—or dress down—your core pieces. Pack nice costume jewelry or scarves instead of your ruby earrings or your grandmother's cameo. The fewer valuables you bring on a trip, the better. The last thing you want to worry about is losing them or having them stolen.

And remember, you can always pick up fun, fresh accessories while you're traveling. Keep your eyes open for local specialties. If you're going to Scotland, look for great bargains in wool. The Far East has great silks, and Africa, wonderful batiks. Leave your pearls at home and pick up some gorgeous shell earrings to wear with your sundress. Which brings me to my final point. Always remember to pack an extra bag when you travel to haul home any goodies you buy on the road!

Hotel Amenities

Try to find out ahead of time what conveniences your hotel offers. Whether you're staying at an expensive hotel or a moderately priced chain, chances are they'll have a blow dryer mounted in the bathroom. You can leave yours behind. Most good hotels come equipped with irons or have them available through room service, so you can leave your travel iron at home, too. Call ahead if you're unsure—the room in your suitcase will be worth the long-distance charge.

How to Measure

Bust: Measure under the arms around the fullest part of the bust

Waist: Measure around the smallest part of the waistline

Hips: Measure around the fullest part of the hips, about 8" below the waist

Women's sizes (in both Misses and Petites) fit a fuller figure in the waist and hips and allow more fabric for comfort in the upper arms and shoulders than Misses sizes.

Since most women are not evenly proportioned, the bust measurement should be used for tops, easy-fitting dresses, and coats; the hip measurement for pants, skirts, and narrow dresses; and the waist measurement for fitted styles.

❋ Petites' Size Range—5' 3" and under

Bust	33.5	34.5	35.5	36.5	38	39.5	41	42.5	44
Waist	24.5	25.5	26.5	27.5	29	30.5	32	33.5	35
Hip	35	36	37	38	39.5	41	42.5	44	45.5
Order size	4	6	8	10	12	14	16	18	20
	X-small	Small		Medium		Large		X-Large	

❋ Misses' Size Range—5' 4" and above

Bust	34	35	36	37	38.5	40	41.5	43	44.5
Waist	25	26	27	28	29.5	31	32.5	34	35.5
Hip	35.5	36.5	37.5	38.5	40	41.5	43	44.5	45.5
Order size	4	6	8	10	12	14	16	18	20
	X-small	Small		Medium		Large		X-Large	

❋ Women's Size Range—5' 4" and above

Bust	44	46	48	50	52	54
Waist	35.5	37.5	39.5	41.5	43.5	45.5
Hip	46	48	50	52	54	56
Order size	18W	20W	22W	24W	26W	28W
	1X		2X		3X	

A Glossary of Fashion Terms

A-line dress dress that flares slightly from the bodice to the hem

A-line skirt skirt that is fitted at the waist and flares slightly

Ascot collar collar with an attached necktie that ties into a bow in front

ballet neckline neckline formed by a slightly curved, wide opening between the two shoulder seams

beading type of embroidery in which beads are sewn onto a fabric; used with dressy sweaters, formal wear, and purses

bell sleeve narrow sleeve that flares into a wide bell-shape at the hem

bell-bottoms pants that flare from the knee to a wide hem

Bermuda shorts straight-legged shorts, knee-length or just above the knee

bike shorts knee-length, skintight shorts; often in Lycra spandex

blouson blouse full blouse gathered into a band at the hemline, either waist-length or hip-length

blouson dress dress with a blouson top that drapes over a low waistline

boat neckline slightly high neckline formed by a straight, wide opening between the two shoulder seams

bolero short jacket or vest that falls at or above the waistline, usually collarless with a rounded front and no fastenings

boot-cut pants straight pants that flare slightly at the hem

cap sleeve not a true, set-in sleeve, but part of a garment that just covers the top of the shoulder when the cut includes an extra amount of fabric at the shoulder seams

Capri pants narrow, midcalf-length pants, usually with a small slit in the outer seam at the hem

City shorts tailored shorts worn in place of a skirt or trousers with a suit jacket

convertible collar collar that can be worn open, like a small notched collar, or closed and turned down when it is fastened at the neck by a small button and loop

cowlneck large draped collar that folds over on itself and extends towards the shoulders

crewneck rounded, collarless neckline that comes up to the collarbone; usually used with knits and finished with ribbing

cuffed sleeve wrist-length sleeve that is set smoothly into the shoulder and ends in a buttoned cuff, often with a pleat or pleats

culottes very wide-legged pants that look like a skirt with a pleat at the center front and back; also called a divided skirt

dirndl slightly full to full skirt gathered at the waistband

dolman sleeve sleeve that tapers down from a wide armhole to a narrow hem, often part of the cut of the bodice rather than set-in

drape neckline a loose wide neckline similar to a boat neckline but with fabric (often bias-cut) draping down in front

duster lightweight, long-length coat or vest with wide shoulders and sleeves, often with large patch-pockets

flutter sleeve flowing short sleeve that drapes in folds over the top of the shoulder or upper arm; often used in evening wear—it may or may not be seamed

grandfather collar standing collar similar to a mandarin collar, but slightly lower and closing with a button

halter dress or top bare-shouldered and low-backed dress or top held up by a fabric piece, a strap, or a string that goes around the neck

handkerchief skirt skirt that falls into a series of even triangular points all around the hemline

hip-huggers pants that fit below the natural waistline, coming only as high as the hips; often worn with a wide belt

jewel neckline rounded neckline that comes to just below the collarbone

keyhole neckline slightly high, rounded neckline that has a shaped notch in the front

leggings skintight knit pants, usually with an elastic waist

mandarin collar high collar made of a standing band that meets in an open notch at the center

midriff shirt shirt with a hem that ends just below the bustline to reveal the midriff; often in a button-down style that ties under the bust

minidress, miniskirt very short dress or skirt, with a midthigh hemline several inches above the knee

mock-turtleneck collar a high, close-fitting collar made by stitching a flat band around the circumference of a garment's neckline to imitate a turtleneck

notched collar a collar that forms a notch where it attaches to the lapels of a garment

pashmina an oversize, rectangular scarf worn as a wrap, traditionally made of goat's wool but available in a range of fabrics

pedal pushers straight-legged pants that end either just below the knee or midcalf

pencil skirt flat-front skirt that fits smoothly over the hips and then narrows, with a hemline just below the knee

pleated trousers trousers with front pleats and either straight or tapered legs

puff sleeve short sleeve gathered into a cuff to form a high, rounded puff-shape

Queen Anne collar high collar that stands up at the back and sides with the two points touching the chin in front

raglan sleeve sleeve that is set in with diagonal seams that slant up from the bottom of the armhole to the neckline

running shorts loose athletic shorts, usually with an elastic or drawstring waist

sarong skirt made of a large piece of fabric that wraps around the body and tucks or ties at the waist

scoop neckline rounded neckline cut deeply in the front or the back and the front

shawl collar soft, notchless collar made of a single cut of fabric that folds over on itself in a curve that follows the front opening of the garment

sheath straight, slightly fitted dress usually with vertical darts and a hemline that falls at or just above the knee

short sleeve sleeve that ends at or above the elbow

Skort® miniskirt over an attached pair of shorts; also called a scooter skirt

slim skirt straight skirt that fits smoothly over the hips, knee-length or just above or below the knee

spaghetti strap thin, often rounded, fabric strap that goes over the shoulder on a bare-shouldered top or dress

square neckline straight neckline with squared corners

stirrup pants narrow pants with a band of elastic at the bottom of each leg, which is worn under the foot and inside the shoe

stovepipe pants straight, narrow-legged pants

tank top sleeveless top with ample armholes and a rounded neckline in front and back, forming wide straps over the shoulders

three-quarter sleeve sleeve that ends midway between the elbow and wrist

trumpet skirt straight skirt with a flared flounce at the hem

tulip skirt gathered skirt that swells out from the waistline and then tapers in at the hem; also called a bubble skirt

tunic jacket straight, loose-fitting jacket, usually hip- or thigh-length

turtleneck collar a high, close-fitting collar made by folding the garment's fabric back over itself around the circumference of the neck; usually used with knits

tuxedo jacket straight, shawl-collared jacket with a one-button closing, modeled on the traditional jacket of man's formal tuxedo

V-neck neckline that forms a V-shape, ending anywhere from the collarbone to between the breasts

wing collar 1. tailored collar of a button-front shirt that ends in spreading points. 2. tailored collar ending in two tightly folded-over points; the traditional collar worn with a man's tuxedo

wraparound skirt skirt that wraps around the body and fastens with a button or tie at the waist

Index

Acknowledgements

Most importantly, I would like to thank my QVC viewers for their continued loyalty and support. Their enthusiasm pushes me forward and keeps me going.

I dedicate this book to my loving husband Richard who has brought great joy to my life. He stands behind me at all times and puts everything into perspective for me. His intelligence, understanding, and persistent devotion are unsurpassed. I also dedicate this book to my three wonderful children Michael, David, and Jaclyn who keep me grounded and make all my hard work worthwhile.

A big hug and an enormous thank you to Audrey Graver who has always encouraged me both professionally and personally. I am grateful to have the best mother-in-law, friend, and design talent imaginable.

To my mother, Shirley Hecht whose love and support gave me the confidence to trust my instincts—thank you for always being there for me and for believing in me.

I am especially grateful to Darlene Daggett for her support and wisdom. And of course, to Doug Briggs for making this possible for everyone involved.

A big thank you to all my friends and talented merchants at QVC: Bob Ayd, Terry Heyman, Chris Morley, Melanie Nelson, Cindy Derkacz, Michele Okuniewski, and MaryKay DeZura. Also, thanks to Vera Shelton Fairbanks who first brought my line to QVC. To Pat DeMentri, a heartfelt thanks for both your talent and your friendship. And a huge thank you to all the other terrific hosts I've had the pleasure of working with at QVC.

A very special thank you to all the people who played an important role in the creation and production of this book at QVC Publishing: Jill Cohen and her associates Sarah Butterworth and Cassandra Reynolds.

I am also grateful to my writer, Sheri Holman, and talented illustrator, Mary Lynn Blasutta.

Thank you to Bob Winer and Mike Glass at Winer Industries who work very hard to produce my line and maintain my standards of excellence.

And lastly, I want to thank all the exceptional people that work in production and order entry at QVC—without them none of this would ever happen.

Final Thoughts

It's me—Susan. You know me from my television show and now that you've read my book, you know that I'm an artist at heart. But what you may not realize is that I am also a hard-working designer, business woman, wife, and mother. I'm fortunate enough to love the work that I do both in business and at home. I make the most of every moment and I take nothing for granted. I know first-hand how tough it can be to be everything to everyone, to get a thousand things done (hopefully), make all those appointments, take care of the kids, rush off to dinner. . . and still look your best.

Life can be challenging—dressing should not be. I hope my book has inspired you and has given you some insight into how to build your own confident wardrobe, so that no matter where you're dashing off to, you have that extra spring in your step that comes from knowing that your clothes are working for you.